T0226719

Management of Acute and Chronic Headache Pain

Editor

STEVEN D. WALDMAN

MEDICAL CLINICS OF NORTH AMERICA

www.medical.theclinics.com

March 2013 • Volume 97 • Number 2

ELSEVIER

1600 John F. Kennedy Boulevard • Suite 1800 • Philadelphia, Pennsylvania, 19103-2899

http://www.theclinics.com

MEDICAL CLINICS OF NORTH AMERICA Volume 97, Number 2
March 2013 ISSN 0025-7125, ISBN-13: 978-1-4557-7118-9

Editor: Pamela Hetherington

Medical Clinics of North America (ISSN 0025-7125) is published bimonthly by Elsevier Inc., 360 Park Avenue South, New York, NY 10010-1710. Months of issue are January, March, May, July, September, and November. Periodicals postage paid at New York, NY, and additional mailing offices. Subscription prices are USD 241 per year for US individuals, USD 441 per year for US institutions, USD 121 per year for US students, USD 307 per year for Canadian individuals, USD 572 per year for Canadian institutions, USD 190 per year for Canadian students, USD 372 per year for international individuals, USD 572 per year for international institutions and USD 190 per year for international students. To receive student/resident rate, orders must be accompanied by name of affiliated institution, date of term, and the *signature* of program/residency coordinator on institution letterhead. Orders will be billed at individual rate until proof of status is received. Foreign air speed delivery is included in all *Clinics* subscription prices. All prices are subject to change without notice. **POSTMASTER:** Send address changes to *Medical Clinics of North America*, Elsevier Health Sciences Division, Subscription Customer Service, 3251 Riverport Lane, Maryland Heights, MO 63043. **Customer Service: Telephone: 1-800-654-2452** (U.S. and Canada); **1-314-447-8871** (outside U.S. and Canada). **Fax: 1-314-447-8029. E-mail: journalscustomerservice-usa@elsevier.com** (for print support); **journalsonlinesupport-usa@ elsevier.com** (for online support).

Reprints. For copies of 100 or more of articles in this publication, please contact the Commercial Reprints Department, Elsevier Inc., 360 Park Avenue South, New York, NY 10010-1710. Tel.: 212-633-3812; Fax: 212-462-1935; E-mail: reprints@elsevier.com.

Medical Clinics of North America is also published in Spanish by McGraw-Hill Interamericana Editores S. A., P.O. Box 5-237, 06500 Mexico, D.F., Mexico.

Medical Clinics of North America is covered in *MEDLINE/PubMed (Index Medicus)*, *Current Contents, ASCA, Excerpta Medica, Science Citation Index, and ISI/BIOMED.*

Printed and bound by CPI Group (UK) Ltd, Croydon, CR0 4YY

Transferred to digital print 2012

PROGRAM OBJECTIVE

The goal of *Medical Clinics of North America* is to keep practicing physicians up to date with current clinical practice by providing timely articles reviewing the state of the art in patient care.

TARGET AUDIENCE

All practicing physicians and other healthcare professionals.

LEARNING OBJECTIVES

Upon completion of this activity, participants should be able to:

1. Review the management and treatment of headaches from the following origins: Cervicogenic; Ocular and Periocular; ear, nose, throat and sinus.
2. Describe the use of laboratory testing and imaging in the evaluation of headaches.
3. Recall the use of physical examination to better manage acute and chronic headache pain.

ACCREDITATION

The Elsevier Office of Continuing Medical Education (EOCME) is accredited by the Accreditation Council for Continuing Medical Education (ACCME) to provide continuing medical education for physicians.

The EOCME designates this journal-based CME activity for a maximum of 11 *AMA PRA Category 1 Credit*(s)™. Physicians should claim only the credit commensurate with the extent of their participation in the activity.

All other health care professionals completing continuing education credit for this activity will be issued a certificate of participation.

DISCLOSURE OF CONFLICTS OF INTEREST

The EOCME assesses conflict of interest with its instructors, faculty, planners, and other individuals who are in a position to control the content of CME activities. All relevant conflicts of interest that are identified are thoroughly vetted by EOCME for fair balance, scientific objectivity, and patient care recommendations. EOCME is committed to providing its learners with CME activities that promote improvements or quality in healthcare and not a specific proprietary business or a commercial interest.

The planning committee, staff, authors and editors listed below have identified no financial relationships or relationships to products or devices they or their spouse/life partner have with commercial interest related to the content of this CME activity:

Bernard M. Abrams, MD; Stephanie Carter; Nicole Congleton; Charles D. Donohoe, MD; Sandra Lavery; Malisa S. Lester, MD; Benjamin P. Liu, MD; Jill B. McNair; Santha Priya; Maunak V. Rana, MD; Stephen D. Silberstein, MD; Nailia Vodovskaia, MD; Steven D. Waldman, MD, JD; Corey W. Waldman, MD; Jennifer E. Waldman; and Reid A. Waldman.

The planning committee, staff, authors and editors listed below have identified financial relationships or relationships to products or devices they or their spouse/life partner have with commercial interest related to the content of this CME activity:

Frederick Freitag, DO has participated on the speakers bureau and as a consultant for Allergan and Zogenix; and speakers bureau for Nautilus.

UNAPPROVED/OFF-LABEL USE DISCLOSURE

The EOCME requires CME faculty to disclose to the participants:

1. When products or procedures being discussed are off-label, unlabelled, experimental, and/or investigational (not US Food and Drug Administration (FDA) approved); and
2. Any limitations on the information presented, such as data that are preliminary or that represent ongoing research, interim analyses, and/or unsupported opinions. Faculty may discuss information about pharmaceutical agents that is outside of FDA-approved labelling. This information is intended solely for CME and is not intended to promote off-label use of these medications. If you have any questions, contact the medical affairs department of the manufacturer for the most recent prescribing information.

TO ENROLL

To enroll in the *Medical Clinics of North America* Continuing Medical Education program, call customer service at 1-800-654-2452 or sign up online at http://www.theclinics.com/home/cme. The CME program is available to subscribers for an additional annual fee of USD $267.

METHOD OF PARTICIPATION

In order to claim credit, participants must complete the following:

1. Complete enrolment as indicated above.
2. Read the activity.
3. Complete the CME Test and Evaluation. Participants must achieve a score of 70% on the test. All CME Tests and Evaluations must be completed online.

CME INQUIRIES/SPECIAL NEEDS

For all CME inquiries or special needs, please contact elsevierCME@elsevier.com.

MEDICAL CLINICS OF NORTH AMERICA

FORTHCOMING ISSUES

May 2013
Early Diagnosis and Intervention in Predementia Alzheimer's Disease
Jose Molinuevo, Jeffrey Cummings, Bruno Dubois, and Philip Scheltens, *Editors*

July 2013
The Diabetic Foot
Andrew Boulton, *Editor*

September 2013
Infectious Disease Threats
Douglas Paauw, *Editor*

RECENT ISSUES

January 2013
Diabetic Chronic Kidney Disease
Mark E. Williams, MD, FACP, FASN, *Editor*

November 2012
Interventions in Infectious Disease Emergencies
Nancy Misri Khardori, MD, PhD, FACP, FIDSA, *Editor*

July 2012
Chronic Obstructive Pulmonary Disease
Stephen I. Rennard, MD, and Bartolome R. Celli, MD, *Editors*

RELATED INTEREST

Medical Clinics of North America, Volume 94, Issue 5 (September 2010)
Otolaryngology for the Internist
Matthew Ryan, *Editor*

Contributors

EDITOR

STEVEN D. WALDMAN, MD, JD
Clinical Professor of Anesthesiology, School of Medicine, University of Missouri-Kansas City, Kansas City, Missouri

AUTHORS

BERNARD M. ABRAMS, MD
Clinical Professor of Neurology, School of Medicine, University of Missouri-Kansas City, Kansas City, Missouri

CHARLES D. DONOHOE, MD
Neurologist, Associate Clinical Professor of Neurology, School of Medicine, University of Missouri-Kansas City, Independence, Missouri

FREDERICK FREITAG, DO
Medical Director, Department of Neurosciences, Baylor University Medical Center, Dallas, Texas

MALISA S. LESTER, MD
Instructor of Radiology, Section of Neuroradiology, Department of Radiology, Northwestern Memorial Hospital, Feinberg School of Medicine of Northwestern University, Chicago, Illinois

BENJAMIN P. LIU, MD
Assistant Professor of Radiology, Section of Neuroradiology, Department of Radiology, Northwestern Memorial Hospital, Feinberg School of Medicine of Northwestern University, Chicago, Illinois

MAUNAK V. RANA, MD
Medical Director, Chicago Anesthesia Pain Specialists; Department of Anesthesiology, Director of Pain Management, Advocate Illinois Masonic Medical Center, Clinical Assistant Professor of Anesthesiology, University of Illinois-Chicago, Chicago, Illinois

STEPHEN D. SILBERSTEIN, MD
Professor of Neurology, Jefferson Medical College, Thomas Jefferson University; Director, Jefferson Headache Center, Philadelphia, Pennsylvania

NAILIA VODOVSKAIA, MD
Jefferson Headache Center, Philadelphia, Pennsylvania

COREY W. WALDMAN, MD
Krieger Eye Institute at Sinai Hospital, Baltimore, Maryland

JENNIFER E. WALDMAN
Brain Tissue Bank, School of Medicine, University of Missouri-Kansas City, Kansas City, Missouri

REID A. WALDMAN
Free Eye Clinic, School of Medicine, University of Missouri-Kansas City, Kansas City, Missouri

STEVEN D. WALDMAN, MD, JD
Clinical Professor of Anesthesiology, School of Medicine, University of Missouri-Kansas City, Kansas City, Missouri

Contents

> The targeted headache history is paramount in the diagnosis of headache and facial pain. Through placing symptoms in categories, a clear picture of the headache diagnosis will begin to emerge. The physical examination yields no positive findings in most patients with headache. Medication overuse headache is emerging as a common reason for inability to control headaches.

> The most critical element in headache evaluation is the history. The targeted history differentiates primary from secondary headaches and provides a realistic list of conditions associated with secondary headache. Several of these conditions present with specific physical findings, such as papilledema, Horner's syndrome, or a cranial nerve palsy. The targeted physical examination of the patient with headache takes less than 3 minutes. The ability to recognize a few straightforward clinical findings directs the evaluation in the proper direction.

> Blood tests have a minor role in headache management and that role is limited to a few secondary headache conditions. In headache, as with any symptom, laboratory tests should be chosen based on solid clues derived from the targeted history and physical examination. A shotgun approach to blood tests that includes rare diseases or those with low local prevalence frequently yields false-positive results, which exposes the patient to the expense, anxiety, and risk inherent in misdiagnosis. Keep it simple and do not forget about spinal fluid.

> Headaches can be benign or life threatening but, with careful attention to the details described in this article, the correct diagnosis and treatment can be arrived at in many cases. Modern imaging techniques have taken the guesswork out of many conditions but a high index of suspicion and attention to red flags helps avoid potential adverse outcomes in headache encounters in a high proportion of cases.

should also remain vigilant for diseases of this anatomic region that do not cause pain but have the potential, if undiagnosed, to create significant problems for the patient, such as acoustic neuroma, thyroid carcinoma, and malignant melanoma. This article provides the clinician with a concise road map for the evaluation of painful conditions of the ear, nose, sinuses, and throat that may be responsible for headache.

Trigeminal autonomic cephalalgias are short-lasting primary headache disorders associated with autonomic symptoms. Paroxysmal hemicrania is a rare headache disorder similar to cluster headache. Short-lasting unilateral neuralgiform headache attacks with conjunctival injection and tearing (SUNCT) and short-lasting unilateral neuralgiform headache attacks with cranial autonomic symptoms (SUNA) are unusual headache syndromes typified by a high frequency of severe, brief, unilateral attacks that usually occur in the distribution of the trigeminal nerve. SUNCT is a subtype of SUNA in which both conjunctival injection and tearing are present. SUNA differs from SUNCT in that autonomic symptoms are less prominent.

Giant cell arteritis is one of the most serious medical emergencies encountered in the practice of ophthalmology because it may result in loss of vision in one or both eyes. This vision loss is preventable if patients are diagnosed early and treated immediately with high doses of corticosteroids.

Overuse of any class of drugs, Triptans, ergots, opioids, simple, or combination analgesics used to treat acute headaches, especially migraine, can lead to the development of medication overuse headache. People suffering from primary headache types, such as migraine or tension-type headache, are at higher risk to develop chronic headache following the overuse of acute headache drugs. Treatment of medication overuse headache requires withdrawal as an initial step, coincident initiation of preventive treatment, a multidisciplinary setting, and includes education of patients.

Preface

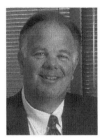

Steven D. Waldman, MD, JD
Editor

All scholarly writings on headache begin with a variation on the same theme:

- Headaches are the most common neurologic complaint seen by physicians
- Headaches are a universal human condition
- Every patient has suffered from headache at some time in their life.

Given that these statements are true, one must wonder why a disease as common as headache creates so much stress, anxiety, and frustration for the treating physician and patient alike? I suspect that there are 2 reasons the complaint of headache evokes these negative emotions in many physicians and virtually all headache patients: the first reason is that the vast majority of patients suffering from headache have completely normal physical examinations and laboratory and neuroimaging evaluations. The clinician faced with a patient whose headaches are poorly controlled is constantly wondering how a patient who has no objective evidence of disease can take up so much time and energy and create so much stress, anxiety, and frustration? Not surprisingly, the patient is wondering the same thing. How can I be "normal" when this headache hurts so bad?

This brings us to reason number 2. At the back of both the treating physician's and the headache sufferer's mind is the nagging worry that something "has been missed" and that the patient's headache is the harbinger of a life-threatening illness, because both the lay public and the physician know that headaches can spell big trouble: brain tumors, strokes, aneurysms, and/or meningitis. Ignoring or trivializing the complaint of headache is to flirt with disaster. Many physicians, especially many physicians in my specialty of pain management, simply refuse to treat patients suffering from headache; others immediately refer headache patients to neurologists or other headache specialists, and many prescribe narcotics, the current solution for any and all pain complaints. For the rest of us who continue to treat patients with headache, might I suggest 2 strategies to reduce the stress, anxiety, and frustration. The first strategy is to understand why headache treatment fails and second strategy is to understand what the clinician can do to avoid these headache treatment failures.

Med Clin N Am 97 (2013) xi–xii
http://dx.doi.org/10.1016/j.mcna.2012.12.011
0025-7125/13/$ – see front matter © 2013 Published by Elsevier Inc.

medical.theclinics.com

Headache treatment fails for one or more of the following reasons:

1. The diagnosis is incorrect (every bad headache is a migraine fallacy)
2. The diagnosis is incomplete (the patient has more than one type of headache, see number 1)
3. Medication overuse abounds yet is underdiagnosed (especially opioids in our current environment of opioid as the panacea for all that ails the world)
4. Headache triggers are ignored (especially caffeine, wine, and HRT)
5. Medication misadventures (including too much too early, too little too late, wrong drug due to wrong diagnosis, abortive rather than preventative, drugs prone to cause rebound headache, and, of course, noncompliance)
6. Failure to identify comorbid conditions (the MRI was normal, but I didn't take a blood pressure)
7. Psychosocial issues

The first step is to be aware of these pitfalls and to look for them constantly in your treatment plan that has gone awry. Second, play the numbers. Common headaches are common, and rare headaches are rare. Your starting point when approaching any headache patient is to rule out the Big Four: tension-type headache, medication overuse headache, migraine, and cluster. Third, follow your gut. If you think the patient is sick, pull out all the stops. This is not the time to watch and wait. Fourth, don't fall in love with a diagnosis or a test result. If things aren't getting better, rethink the diagnosis, and if things move from the "well" to "sick" scenario, repeat everything: the history, physical exam, the lab work, and, most importantly, the neuroimaging.

It is my strong belief that if you follow these common sense steps, steps followed by all good physicians, your comfort level with headache will improve as will your patient care!

Steven D. Waldman, MD, JD
11600 Manor
Leawood, KS 66211, USA

E-mail address:
sdwaldmanmd@gmail.com

Targeted Headache History

Steven D. Waldman, MD, JD

KEYWORDS

- Tension-type headache • Migraine with aura • Migraine without aura
- Cluster headache • Trigeminal neuralgia • Targeted headache history

KEY POINTS

- The targeted headache history is paramount in the diagnosis of headache and facial pain.
- Through placing symptoms in categories, a clear picture of the headache diagnosis will begin to emerge.
- The physical examination yields no positive findings in most patients with headache.
- Medication overuse headache is emerging as a common reason for inability to control headaches.

It has been said that if one only has 30 minutes to spend evaluating a patient with headache, 29 minutes should be spent taking a history and 1 minute should be devoted to the physical examination. The reason is that in most patients who present with headache, the diagnosis is made based on information obtained during a targeted headache history rather than from findings gleaned from the physical examination.[1,2] The targeted headache history is crucial for enabling clinicians to sort out the myriad overlapping symptoms associated with headache into discrete groups of symptoms. Through the constellation of symptoms contained in these discrete groups, clinicians are able to paint a clear picture of what each patient's headache symptoms look like and arrive at the most likely diagnosis. Furthermore, the presence of certain symptoms within these discrete groups allows clinicians to more easily identify factors that cause concern and take immediate appropriate action (**Tables 1** and **2**).

Failure to obtain a targeted headache history can lead not only to the implementation of an ineffective treatment plan because the diagnosis is incorrect ("after all everyone knows that any bad headache is a migraine") but also, in some situations, to the failure to recognize life-threatening disease. In simplistic terms, the targeted headache history allows treating clinicians to determine sick from well when evaluating a patient with headaches. If the patient is determined in all probability to be well (ie, has no life-threatening illness), the workup and treatment plan may proceed at a more conservative pace. If, however, the targeted headache history indicates a life-threatening disease process, an aggressive course of action is indicated.

School of Medicine, University of Missouri-Kansas City, 2411 Holmes, Kansas City, MO 64108, USA
E-mail address: sdwaldmanmd@gmail.com

Med Clin N Am 97 (2013) 185–195
http://dx.doi.org/10.1016/j.mcna.2012.12.001
medical.theclinics.com

Table 1
Overlapping symptoms of common headache and facial pain syndromes: pain

Pain	Tension-Type	Migraine Without Aura	Migraine With Aura	Cluster	Trigeminal Neuralgia	Atypical Facial Pain
Severe		X	X	X	X	
Dull	X					X
Throbbing		X	X			
Nonthrobbing	X				X	X
Shock or jab-like				X	X	
Tightness	X					X

Before taking a targeted headache history, clinicians should remember 2 facts: (1) most headaches, although extremely painful and disruptive to the patient, are not life-threatening, and (2) tension-type headache, migraine, and medication overuse headaches constitute more than 90% of headaches encountered in clinical practice.[2] The implications of these facts are obvious: that life-threatening causes of headache are extremely rare, and that the frequency of headache types other than the 3 aforementioned headaches are also rare. These facts make things much easier for those caring for patients presenting with headache by really highlighting symptom groupings that fall outside the expected symptom groupings for the most common types of headache.

When taking the targeted headache history, several areas of historical information should be explored, not only to distinguish the sick patient from the well one but also to attempt to ascertain the specific diagnosis (**Box 1**).

CHRONICITY

The length of illness sets the direction of the initial history and carries much weight in determining sick patients from those who are well. Therefore, it serves as the starting point for the targeted headache history. In general, headaches that have been present for 20 to 30 years are in and of themselves not associated with progressive and life-threatening neurologic disease. This finding leads one to strongly consider the

Table 2
Overlapping symptoms of common headache and facial pain syndromes: location

Pain	Tension-Type	Migraine Without Aura	Migraine With Aura	Cluster	Trigeminal Neuralgia	Atypical Facial Pain
Unilateral		X	X	X	X	X
Bilateral	X				Rare	
Temporal		X	X	X		
Frontal	X	X	X			
Occipital	X	X	X			
Cervical spine	X					X
Ocular				X	X	
Cheek					X	X

Box 1
A suggested framework for the targeted headache history

- Chronicity of headaches
- Age of onset
- Duration of headaches
- Frequency of headaches
- Onset-to-peak time
- Location
- Character of pain
- Severity of pain
- Premonitory symptoms and aurae
- Associated symptoms
- Environmental factors
- Family history
- Pregnancy and menstruation
- Past medical and surgical history
- Past treatments
- Previous diagnostic tests

patient's headache a pain syndrome that should not be associated with loss of life or limb; hence, the well determination is made. This determination sets the tone for the pace and scope of the evaluation and course of treatment. Conversely, the sudden onset of severe headache or the sudden change in the character of a headache pattern that has been stable for many years pushes clinicians to strongly consider that the patient must be placed into the category of sick until proven otherwise. This type of pain manifestation has often been called the *first or worst syndrome*.[3] Patients who fall into this category deserve a high level of scrutiny, and their pain complaint should be viewed as a harbinger of a medical emergency (**Box 2**).

Box 2
Factors that cause concern

- New headache of recent onset ("the first")
- New headache of unusual severity ("the worst")
- Headache associated with neurologic dysfunction
- Headache associated with systemic illness
- Headaches that peak rapidly
- Headaches associated with exertion
- Focal headache
- Sudden change in a previously stable headache pattern
- Headaches associated with the Valsalva maneuver
- Nocturnal headache

Pitfalls when taking the chronicity portion of the targeted headache history include (1) failing to identify ominous changes in a longstanding stable headache or facial pain syndrome, (2) attributing the sudden onset of symptoms to a benign cause without adequate evaluation (eg, attributing a sudden severe headache in a patient with generalized staphylococcal sepsis simply to fever without ruling out cerebral abscess), and (3) failing to recognize new symptoms superimposed on chronic headache symptoms (eg, attributing increased headache when coughing to a patient's chronic cervical spondylotic disease while ignoring the fact that the patient also has known breast malignancy, which could silently metastasize to the brain, causing increased intracranial pressure).[4]

AGE AT ONSET

Headaches that begin in childhood through the second decade of life are most often vascular in nature. Headache pain that begins later in life is statistically most commonly tension-type or from medication overuse, although both can occur in younger populations.[2] Two notable exceptions to this rule are trigeminal neuralgia, which is rarely seen before the third decade of life unless in association with multiple sclerosis and giant cell arteritis, the incidence of which increases markedly during the fifth and sixth decades[5,6] (see article written by Waldman et al, elsewhere in this issue).

Pitfalls in the age-at-onset portion of the targeted history center around 2 facts:

1. As one gets older, the chances of systemic illness such as hypertension, glaucoma, stroke, and cancer increase.
2. Children, adolescents, and young adults can all experience these systemic illnesses, albeit rarely. Unfortunately, from the point of view of chronologic age, these less common systemic diseases are rarely suspected in this younger age group.

DURATION AND FREQUENCY OF PAIN

The duration and frequency of the patient's headache symptoms may provide clinicians with the best clues as to the classification and diagnosis of the headache. Although most headache and facial pain syndromes occur in a seemingly random and sporadic pattern, careful questioning often reveals an identifiable pattern to aid in the diagnosis. A headache diary kept by the patient for 2 to 3 months may be useful to elucidate an identifiable pattern in difficult or confusing cases.

In general, vascular headaches and trigeminal neuralgia tend to occur in an episodic fashion, with the duration of pain ranging from minutes in the case of cluster headache and trigeminal neuralgia to hours in the case of migraine.[5] Cluster headache may be seasonal, with peak occurrences in the spring and fall.[5,7] Headaches of organic origin (eg, ocular disease, sinus disease, brain tumor) tend to be continuous, with acute exacerbation caused by exercise, change in position, and the Valsalva maneuver. These headache syndromes will worsen over time if the underlying organic disease is not correctly diagnosed and treated or if the disease does not resolve spontaneously. Pain that is present on a daily basis and persists for months to years most likely falls under the category of tension-type headache or medication-overuse headache, or is one of the rarely occurring types of chronic daily headache, such as hemicrania continua.[8]

ONSET-TO-PEAK TIME

When coupled with the frequency and duration portion of the targeted headache history, the onset-to-peak time may help further narrow the diagnostic possibilities

(**Fig. 1**). A rapid onset-to-peak time (seconds to minutes) should increase suspicion of organic disease. Of particular concern are headaches that worsen with activities such as exercise, the Valsalva maneuver, and bending forward (see **Box 2**). Notable exceptions to this rule are cluster headache and trigeminal neuralgia.

Migraine without aura tends to evolve over several hours, with a painless prodrome of premonitory symptoms followed by pain.[9] In the patient who experiences migraine with aura, the headache pain is preceded by promontory symptoms and painless neurologic dysfunction, called *aura*.[5,10] Cluster headache has a much more rapid onset-to–peak time. Tension-type headache pain tends to evolve over a period of hours to days and then remains constant.

Pitfalls when drawing conclusions regarding the onset-to-peak time of a headache or facial pain syndrome include the special situation in which a syndrome with slow onset-to-peak time (eg, tension-type headache) may trigger a syndrome with a more rapid onset-to-peak time (eg, migraine), producing the coexistent or mixed headache syndrome.[11]

Location

The location of headache or facial pain may provide clinicians with additional information for the classification and diagnosis of the patient's pain syndrome. Pain localized to an anatomic structure should be evaluated in the context of common disease entities for that structure (eg, glaucoma, otitis media, dental pain).

The pain of vascular headache is usually unilateral, although the side may change from attack to attack. Cluster headache pain is usually localized to the ocular and retroocular region, whereas migraine tends to involve the entire hemicranium.

Tension-type headache pain is typically bilateral but can be unilateral, often involving the frontal, temporal, and occipital regions. The pain may manifest as bandlike or caplike tightness in the aforementioned anatomic areas. Neck symptoms often coexists in patients experiencing tension-type headache, and may confuse the clinical picture. Trigeminal neuralgia generally involves only one division of the trigeminal nerve (>98%).[5] If the localization of pain overlaps anatomic distribution, nonneuralgic atypical facial pain, referred pain, or local pathologic condition is a more likely explanation.

Pitfalls in assessing location include referred pain and sudden changes of anatomic localization during an attack. Special attention should be given to any typical manifestation or poorly localized pain, because pain referred from tumors of the hypopharynx

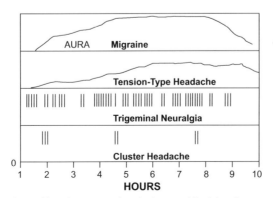

Fig. 1. Onset to peak profile of common headaches and facial pains.

and posterior fossa can easily be misdiagnosed. Pain that is occipital or unilateral but becomes holocranial during the Valsalva maneuver suggests intracranial abnormalities and probable increased intracranial pressure.

CHARACTER AND SEVERITY OF PAIN

Although these symptoms overlap considerably, some generalizations can be made when taking a targeted headache history. Vascular headaches tend to be throbbing and pulsatile in nature, with the pain intensity often described as intense. Cluster headache may have a deeper boring and burning quality. The pain of cluster headache is reputed to be among the worst pains known to mankind. Trigeminal neuralgia is typically described as paroxysmal jab-like or shock-like pain, in contradistinction to non-neuralgic atypical facial pain, which is more often a dull ache and nagging in character.[5] Tension-type headache is a persistent dull aching pain that is often described as band-like or vice-like, with a constant baseline level of pain and occasional severe exacerbations. Headache associated with lumbar puncture will worsen when the patient assumes the recumbent position.

Pitfalls in judging the character of pain include the fact that the patient may experience more than one type of headache and that the most recent or most severe headache may be the one that the patient best remembers, even though it is not the most common type for that patient. This scenario is seen frequently in patients with coexistent or mixed headaches with a predominant tension-type component.[11]

PREMONITORY SYMPTOMS AND AURAE

Premonitory symptoms and aurae are usually associated with vascular headaches, specifically migraine. Premonitory symptoms usually precede the migraine attack by 2 to 48 hours. Among the common premonitory symptoms experienced with migraine are fatigue, elation, depression, changes in libido, craving for certain foods, and abnormal hunger. These premonitory symptoms occur before an attack of migraine without aura (previously called *common migraine*) or before the onset of aura associated with an attack of migraine with aura (previously called *classic migraine*).

Aurae are manifested by focal cerebral dysfunction. Most aurae are ocular symptoms originating in the visual cortex of the occipital lobe (**Fig. 2**).[10] They are presumably caused by localized ischemia of this anatomic region. Other examples of aurae include disturbances of smell, feeling, or motor function.

Pitfalls encountered include the fact that many people who experience chronic headache may adopt symptoms associated with chronic headaches other than the type they experience. These symptoms are gleaned from articles in the lay press and from repeated visits to health care professionals in an attempt to find relief. One can easily imagine how patients would feel obligated to report associated sensitivity to light or nausea after being repeatedly asked about these symptoms by the various physicians they see. The acceptance of these symptoms at face value by a physician may lead to an erroneous diagnosis. Tumors involving the occipital lobe may produce symptoms similar to migrainous aura (**Fig. 3**).[12] These symptoms are usually more persistent relative to those associated with migraine with aura, and careful questioning may help identify symptoms that indicate a structural lesion (**Box 3**).

ASSOCIATED SYMPTOMS

The targeted history should include questions regarding other symptoms. Photophobia, sonophobia, nausea, vomiting, aversion to strong odors, and focal neurologic

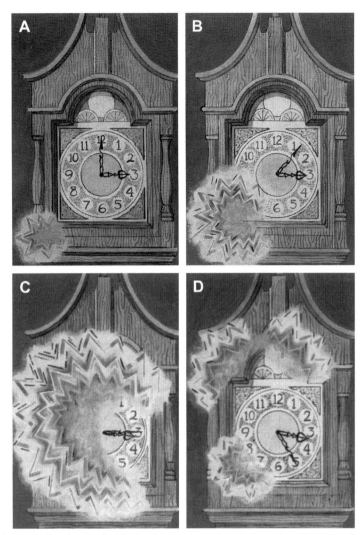

Fig. 2. Classical migrainous scintillating scotoma march and expansion of fortification figures. Initial small paracentral scotoma (*A*). Enlarging scotoma 7 minutes later (*B*). Scotoma obscuring much of central vision 15 minutes later (*C*). Break up of scotoma at 20 minutes (*D*). (*From* Hupp SL, Kline LB, Corbett JJ. Visual disturbances of migraine. Surv Ophthalmol 1989;33(4):221–36.)

changes may be seen with migraine.[5,11] These symptoms may also be seen with other headache and facial pain syndromes. Cluster headache is frequently accompanied by symptoms of complete or partial Horner syndrome, including lacrimation, heavy rhinorrhea, and blanching of the face on the affected side.[5,7]

Meningeal signs will occur rapidly after onset of subarachnoid hemorrhage, as will the focal neurologic changes of stroke. Tinnitus or hearing loss in patients with trigeminal neuralgia may indicate an underlying brainstem tumor.[13] Weakness, bowel or bladder difficulties, and sudden visual loss in patients experiencing trigeminal neuralgia may suggest coexisting multiple sclerosis.

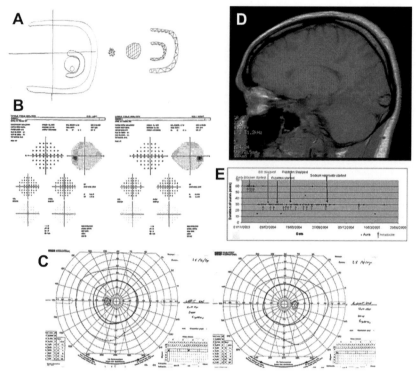

Fig. 3. (*A*) Visual aura experienced by case one. A star shaped pin-point of light appearing in the right lower quadrant of the visual field, expanding first as a circle and then a horse-shoe of triangular zigzag lines over several minutes and occupying the entire right peripheral hemifield over 2 minutes. (*B*) 24-2 Humphrey visual field exam showing a normal visual field in both eyes. (*C*) Goldmann perimetry showing a normal visual field in both eyes. (*D*) T1 weighted sagittal MRI brain scan showing a heterogeneous lesion within the left occipital lobe, with a hemosiderin rim signal intensity, in keeping with a cavernoma. (*E*) Symptom diary showing the frequency of headaches and visual aura over 18 months which were significantly reduced with sodium valproate. (*From* Shams PN, Plant GT, Migraine-like visual aura due to focal cerebral lesions: case series and review. Surv Ophthalmol 2011;56(2):135–61.)

PRECIPITATING FACTORS

Migraine headache may be triggered by change in diet or sleep habits, tyramine-containing foods, monosodium glutamate, nitrates, alcohol, hormones and oral contraceptives, fatigue, stress, menstruation, underlying tension-type headache, strong odors, and bright sunlight.[14,15] Tension-type headache is usually triggered by underlying environmental or physiologic stress, depression, fatigue, and, occasionally, abnormalities of the cervical spine.[14] Like migraine, cluster headache may be triggered by alcohol, high altitude, and, occasionally, vasodilating substances.[5] Nonneuralgic atypical facial pain may be caused by stress, bruxism, prolonged dental work, and, occasionally, poorly fitting dental appliances.[5]

Environmental Factors

Contact with vasodilating substances via diet or absorption through the skin or respiratory tract may precipitate vascular headache. Stress and pressure in the workplace,

> **Box 3**
> **Clinical features differentiating the visual aura of migraine from those of structural cortical lesions**
>
> 1. Clinical features that cannot reliably differentiate the visual aurae of migraine from those caused by structural lesions:
>
>   a. The presence of scintillating scotoma
>
>   b. Duration of visual aura
>
>   c. Visual aura recurring in the same hemifield
>
>   d. Previous history of migraine with or without aura
>
> 2. Clinical features that should raise doubts about a diagnosis of idiopathic migraine:
>
>   a. Absence of headache, especially in patients younger than 50 years
>
>   b. Brief visual aura lasting seconds or less than 5 minutes
>
>   c. Age greater than 40 years, especially without a past history of migraine
>
> 3. Clinical features warranting neuroimaging:
>
>   a. Stereotypical visual aura
>
>   b. Increase in frequency of visual aura
>
>   c. Change in the pattern or characteristics of longstanding visual aura
>
>   d. Any unexplained visual field defect
>
>   e. Negative visual phenomena/subjective persistence of a scotoma after a typical visual aura
>
> *From* Shams PN, Plant GT, Migraine-like visual aura due to focal cerebral lesions: case series and review. Surv Ophthalmol 2011;56(2):135–61.

video display terminals, industrial fumes, carbon monoxide, high altitude, and airborne contaminants carried by heating and cooling systems also have been implicated as precipitating factors for headache.

Family History

Migraine is a familial disease. If both parents experience from migraine, a 70% to 75% chance exists that their children will have migraine.[16] If only one parent has the disease, the incidence in offspring decreases to 45%. Cluster headache, trigeminal neuralgia, and nonneuralgic atypical facial pain do not seem to be hereditary in nature.

A common pitfall encountered when exploring familial history as part of the targeted history is that headache and facial pain may be a learned behavior, which may explain the clustering of people experiencing headache throughout several generations of a given family, even though no heritable basis exists for their disease.

Pregnancy and Menstruation

Migraine may commonly occur with the onset of menses.[17] Pregnancy seems to provide some amelioration of migraine headache after the first trimester. Menopause usually has the same effect; the migraine headache may disappear or decrease markedly in intensity and frequency during and after the climacteric.[18] Hormone replacement therapy given at the time of menopause may prolong the headache syndrome.

Some migraine headaches worsen with the initiation of oral contraceptives. Concerns have been raised that the use of this group of drugs may increase the incidence of stroke in patients who experience migraine and in those who experience focal neurologic symptoms as part of an aura. This risk may be further increased in patients who are smokers. Other forms of contraception usually provide a more favorable risk/benefit ratio in this group of patients; therefore, oral contraceptives should be avoided whenever possible.

A pitfall to avoid is the assumption that all headaches associated with menses are vascular in nature. Many patients may experience a monthly tension-type headache associated with their menses.

Medical/Surgical History

Headache can be a symptom of most systemic illnesses. Specific questioning regarding infection; previous malignancy; the use of medications that may cause headaches (including topical nitroglycerin); trauma; previous cranial surgery; recent lumbar puncture or myelogram; diseases of the eye, ear, nose, throat, and cervical spine; anemia; thyroid disease; travel outside the country; changes in food, sleep, workplace, and job; and, most importantly, environmental stress may reveal important clues.

Past Treatments

Many people with headache have tried various treatment modalities in an effort to obtain pain relief. In evaluating the success or failure of each of these techniques, one may draw a conclusion regarding to the type of treatment likely to be beneficial and the probable diagnosis of the pain syndrome being treated.

Pitfalls when exploring this part of the targeted history center around 3 points:

1. Assessing the adequacy of a trial of a given treatment modality in terms of dosage, duration of treatment, and patient compliance is often impossible.
2. Patients may be using the failure of multiple treatment regimens as a prelude to drug-seeking behavior. This possibility may also be based on the historical finding that the only drugs that have been effective in providing pain relief are controlled substances. This author's strong opinion is that opioids, benzodiazepines, and barbiturates have little if any utility in the treatment of chronic headache and/or facial pain.
3. Medication-overuse headache can blur the classic symptoms of all types of headache, making diagnosis confusing and treatment impossible.

PREVIOUS DIAGNOSTIC TESTS

Physicians must evaluate the adequacy, validity, age, and quality of previous testing when deciding whether additional testing is indicated. Factors that would indicate additional testing include a change in a previously stable headache problem, onset of a new headache, the discovery of a new systemic illness that may be contributing to or causing the pain problem, or new neurologic findings. Clinicians should never completely rely on a negative neuroimaging study in the face of persistent headache, especially in the presence of factors that cause concern.

SUMMARY

Armed with information obtained from the targeted headache history, clinicians can almost always make an accurate diagnosis or at least determine sick from well. Through using the information obtained, clinicians can craft a safe and cost-effective treatment plan that has a high likelihood of success.

REFERENCES

1. Peatfield R. Headache and facial pain. Medicine 2008;36(10):526–30.
2. Bendtsen L, Jensen R. Tension-type headache. Neurol Clin 2009;27(2):525–35.
3. Friedman BW, Lipton RB. Headache emergencies: diagnosis and management. Neurol Clin 2012;30(1):43–59.
4. Kanner R, Argoff CE. Pain management secrets. 3rd edition. Philadelphia: Mosby; 2009.
5. Waldman SD. Atlas of uncommon pain syndromes. 2nd edition. Philadelphia: Saunders; 2008.
6. Cruccu G, Biasiotta A, Di Rezze S, et al. Trigeminal neuralgia and pain related to multiple sclerosis. Pain 2009;143(3):186–91.
7. McGeeney BE. Cluster headache and related disorders. Tech Reg Anesth Pain Manag 2009;13(1):38–41.
8. Antonaci F, Sjaastad O. Hemicrania continua. In: Aminoff MJ, Boller F, Swaab DF, editors. Headache, volume 97: handbook of clinical neurology. Philadelphia: Elsevier; 2010. p. 483–7.
9. Rozen TD. Migraine prodrome: a nose on a face. Lancet 2004;363(9408):517.
10. Foroozan R, Cutrer FM. Transient neurologic dysfunction in migraine. Neurol Clin 2009;27(2):361–78.
11. Thomas SH, Stone CK. Emergency department treatment of migraine, tension, and mixed-type headache. J Emerg Med 1994;12(5):657–64.
12. Shams PN, Plant GT. Migraine-like visual aura due to focal cerebral lesions: case series and review. Surv Ophthalmol 2011;56(2):135–61.
13. Guo Z, Ouyang H, Cheng Z. Surgical treatment of parapontine epidermoid cysts presenting with trigeminal neuralgia. J Clin Neurosci 2011;18(3):344–6.
14. Wöber C, Wöber-Bingöl Ç. Triggers of migraine and tension-type headache. In: Aminoff MJ, Boller F, Swaab DF, editors. Headache, volume 97: handbook of clinical neurology. Philadelphia: Elsevier; 2010. p. 161–72.
15. Zautcke JL, Schwartz JA, Mueller EJ. Chinese restaurant syndrome: a review. Ann Emerg Med 1986;15(10):1210–3.
16. Colson NJ, Lea VA, Quinlan S, et al. The role of vascular and hormonal genes in migraine susceptibility. Mol Genet Metab 2006;88(2):107–13.
17. Marcus DA. Migraine in women. Semin Pain Med 2004;2(2):115–22.
18. Tozer BS, Boatwright EA, David PS, et al. Prevention of migraine in women throughout the life span. Mayo Clin Proc 2006;81(8):1086–92.

The Role of the Physical Examination in the Evaluation of Headache

Charles D. Donohoe, MD

KEYWORDS

- Primary headache • Secondary headaches • Horner's syndrome • Papilledema
- Cranial nerve palsy • Anisocoria • Perineural tumor spread

KEY POINTS

- Physical examination of the patient with headache including mandatory funduscopic examination is often omitted but can easily be performed in less than 3 minutes.
- Horner's syndrome, caused by interruption of the lengthy oculoparasympathetic pathway, is associated with several important causes of secondary headache.
- An acute third nerve palsy with pupillary dilatation suggests aneurysm, and with pupillary sparing suggests diabetes or hypertension; an isolated dilated pupil is not a third nerve palsy.
- Facial numbness CN V combined with facial weakness CN VII should be viewed as a potential red flag for perineural spread of a head and neck malignancy.

INTRODUCTION

Headache is an extremely common complaint and a leading reason for medical consultation. For migraine alone, the prevalence is 17.6% in females and 5.7% in males between the ages of 12 and 80.[1] From a practical standpoint, it makes sense for all medical professionals to be knowledgeable and confident in the management of these patients. Those in clinical practice, whatever the specialty, see patients with headaches.

This article takes a personal perspective. The author, as a practicing neurologist who has been evaluating patients with headache for 35 years, shares his perceptions of the state of the real world of headache including the mistakes, basic principles in evaluation, and what is needed in current clinical practice.

THE CLINICAL PROBLEM DEFINED

A patient with the chief complaint of headaches, particularly those refractory to treatment, is currently in an unfavorable situation. Many practitioners, regardless of

School of Medicine, University of Missouri at Kansas City, 17020 East 40 Highway, Suite 8 Independence, MO 64055, USA
E-mail address: charles.d.donohoe@gmail.com

Med Clin N Am 97 (2013) 197–216
http://dx.doi.org/10.1016/j.mcna.2012.12.010
0025-7125/13/$ – see front matter © 2013 Elsevier Inc. All rights reserved.

medical.theclinics.com

specialty, find the evaluation of these patients to be tedious and unrewarding. Even more unfortunate is that physicians frequently project this lack of interest to the patient. This sets the stage for immediate dissatisfaction and ultimate therapeutic failure. Patients with refractory headaches are also overwhelmed with the massive information on the Internet and are often searching for someone just to take the time and calmly listen to their complaints. This is reasonable in that an efficient and targeted history, in most cases, provides the diagnosis. There is something therapeutic in being able to relate your story to a physician who projects a sincere interest. Finding such a physician in the current medical climate is another matter.

This article considers the targeted physical examination in individuals with headache. This examination is a derivative of the history and is most applicable to the secondary headaches and cranial neuralgias, although objective neurologic findings can be seen with the less common migraine variants seen primarily but not exclusively in young children and adolescents (**Box 1**).[2]

The positive effects of actually physically examining the patient cannot be overstated. In speaking with many patients with headaches over 35 years in neurology, it is remarkable how often they relate that during prior physician encounters their physical examination was entirely omitted. The idea of evaluating a patient with headaches on a regular basis without performing even the fundoscopic examination seems incomprehensible but this does seem to be a common approach.[3]

THE GOAL: A CORRECT DIAGNOSIS

As in the rest of medicine, an accurate headache diagnosis is usually constructed during the history. If the history is concluded without any clear direction as to diagnostic possibilities, the likelihood that the physical examination, laboratory work, or imaging studies will save the day is extremely remote. Most patients with headaches fall into

---

Box 1
Frequently encountered primary headaches and rare migraine variants

Important primary headaches

- Migraine (with and without aura)
- Tension-type headache
- Trigeminal autonomic cephalalgias (cluster headache, paroxysmal hemicrania)
- Primary thunderclap, exertional headache
- Primary cough or stabbing headache
- Hypnic headache
- Hemicrania continua

Migraine variants: present with physical findings

- Hemiplegic migraine: transient hemiparesis, hemiplegia
- Basilar migraine: dysarthria, diplopia, ataxia, disturbance of consciousness
- Childhood periodic syndromes: cyclic vomiting, abdominal pain, vertigo
- Retinal migraine: transient unilateral or bilateral visual loss
- Ophthalmoplegic migraine: migraine followed by cranial nerve (CN) III palsy in children
- Confusional migraine: transient disorientation or encephalopathy in young children

the primary headache category (see **Box 1**). Although patients have long suspected sinus problems, allergies, or a pinched nerve, these are rarely the cause.

Conducting a targeted headache history requires considerable knowledge, experience, and an intuitive sense of recognizing when something just does not fit. Secondary headaches include a long list of conditions, some of which are life-threatening. The real art of headache management is being able to identify those unfortunate individuals who have an extremely common symptom (headache) but a relatively rare cause (**Box 2**). These are patients who are not getting better, who are apprehensive about the accuracy of their diagnosis, and who often shuffle from physician to physician in different specialties. Equally unfortunate is that these complex patients seek care in the emergency room where time constraints and other practicalities place them at additional risk for either misdiagnosis or delayed diagnosis.

They need a medical professional, independent of the letters after their name, experienced and actually interested in headache management who will take the considerable and poorly reimbursed time in reviewing their history, performing the physical examination, obtaining old records, personally examining imaging studies, and pursuing the problem until a correct diagnosis can be formulated. With certain effort and dedication, it usually can. The problem remains that the availability of this selective manpower is inadequate compared with the scope of this common symptom. In the real world, nurse practitioners and physician assistants are increasingly filling this void.

THE PHYSICAL EXAMINATION

In most cases the physical examination of the patient with headache should take less than 3 minutes. Patients are impressed and frequently surprised that they are actually undergoing a physical examination. It should include the following mandatory elements: blood pressure (BP) measurement; assessment of mental status; and CN examination including fundoscopic examination, strength, and gait. In essence, the

---

Box 2
Important causes of secondary headache

Hemorrhage: subarachnoid, epidural, subdural, intraparenchymal, pituitary

Meningitis

Encephalitis

Chiari 1 malformation

Hydrocephalus

Neoplasm

Venous sinus thrombosis

Sphenoid sinusitis

Carotid or vertebral dissection

Idiopathic intracranial hypertension (pseudotumor cerebri)

Low cerebrospinal fluid pressure headache spontaneous/post–lumbar puncture

Temporal (giant cell) arteritis

Carbon monoxide intoxication

Open angle glaucoma

Medication overuse (rebound)

examination is directed by clues obtained during the history. If infection is a consideration, the temperature should be measured.

The integrity of the patient's mental status can usually be assessed during the history and formal testing is reserved only for those with observed defects in speech and cognition. The patient's gait can be monitored by watching them walk from the waiting area. If for some reason you cannot see the optic fundus, do not assume that it is normal. Send the patient to an ophthalmologist who can dilate the pupils and determine if indeed an abnormality is present. Failure to be thorough in this part of the examination can have devastating consequences including permanent visual loss.

The more commonly overlooked secondary headache conditions that I see in my practice include unrecognized idiopathic intracranial hypertension (IIH) (pseudotumor cerebri); Chiari 1 malformation; giant cell (temporal) arteritis; venous sinus thrombosis; acute angle closure glaucoma; carotid and vertebral artery dissection; subdural and subarachnoid hemorrhage (often associated with anticoagulation); and chronic meningitis. A delay in diagnosis of any of these conditions can result in significant medical morbidity and medicolegal exposure.

BP Measurement

BP is very important and should be measured with the patient relaxed and in the sitting position using a conventional manual mercury or aneroid sphygmomanometer. An appropriate cuff size is critical. Although automated oscillometric systems are reasonable alternatives, the BP measurements obtained from these devices are generally lower than those obtained from manual sphygmomanometers.

In 1988 the International Headache Society reached a consensus that mild to moderate degrees of hypertension do not cause headaches.[4] In 2004 they suggested that headache can be caused by severe hypertension associated with pheochromocytoma, hypertensive crisis with and without encephalopathy, preeclampsia and eclampsia, and acute pressor responses to exogenous agents. It is accepted that only severe hypertension, mostly of an acute nature, is a cause of headache.

There is actually a documented inverse relationship between primary headache including tension headache and migraine and BP. In general, BP in patients with primary headache is in the low-normal in range. The phenomenon of hypertension-induced hypalgesia where higher levels of BP inhibit pain transmission through stimulation of baroreceptors possibly interacting through contiguous brainstem nocieceptive and cardiovascular centers has been postulated in headache and a variety of rheumatologic conditions.[5]

Most patients with primary headache disorders have normal to low BP.[6] Only on very rare conditions, where there is an acute and severe elevation of BP (>180/120 mm Hg), is BP believed to be the actual cause of the headache. Although rarely a cause of secondary headaches, hypertension still remains a common disorder (60 million people in the United States) that is frequently unrecognized (30%), totally untreated (40%), or undertreated (67%). These figures are particularly shocking in that BP remains the most important modifiable risk factor for coronary artery disease, stroke, congestive heart failure, end-stage renal disease, and peripheral vascular disease.[7]

In my experience, most patients with tension headache or migraine have low-normal BP. In the rest of my nonheadache practice, about 20% to 30% have hypertension (BP >140/90 mm Hg) that has been either unrecognized or inadequately treated. Although unrelated to headache, the most common, significant, and treatable positive finding on my physical examination is unrecognized or undertreated hypertension. From a public health standpoint, we continue to miss the boat. We are out buying telemedicine robots so that community hospitals can administer tissue plasminogen activator for stroke 25 times a year while millions of patients with inadequately treated hypertension are silently accumulating diffuse atherosclerosis.

Mental Status

The integrity of the patient's mental status is usually determined while taking the history. In elderly individuals who are unaccompanied by a family member or in settings of acute headache, a brief, targeted mental status examination is valuable (**Box 3**). One is testing for deficits in either speech or cognition that would not only be of localizing value but ensure the integrity of the history itself. Although many of the conditions associated with secondary headaches can cause mental status changes, migraine itself is not infrequently associated with cognitive changes of varying degrees.

During the migraine episode there may be changes in the patient's mood in which they become depressed, listless, anxious, or even hostile.[8] During the attack the patient may experience drowsiness, lethargy, or even a state of irresistible somnolence. Migraine can present with major alterations in consciousness, amnesia, hallucinations, and more profound behavioral changes lasting from hours to days. These rare manifestations of confusional or dysphrenic migraine variant can occur at any age but are most common in males during childhood and adolescence.

Headache, if present at all, may be very mild and as such its relationship to migraine may be ignored. These episodic migrainous confusional states are recurrent in up to 25% of individuals. Differential diagnostic considerations include subarachnoid hemorrhage, nonconvulsive status epilepticus, encephalitis, metabolic encephalopathy, and neoplasms. Imaging studies followed by cerebrospinal fluid (CSF) analysis are indicated in the evaluation of the initial presentation.

Subtle changes in mood, behavior, and level of alertness are very common in migraine. More severe and protracted confusional states are very rare but unfortunately are frequently misdiagnosed as either an epileptic or psychiatric event. As is universally the case with misdiagnoses, they often result in considerable social and financial harm to the patient, expose them to the risks of unnecessary medication, and are ultimately extremely difficult to correct. Other neurologic deficits associated with the migraine variants including an oculomotor CN III palsy (ophthalmoplegic migraine), hemiparesis (hemiplegic migraine), ataxia (basilar migraine), and visual loss (retinal migraine) are also prone to misdiagnosis (see **Box 2**).

Cranial Nerve (CN) Examination

The CN examination is an important examination that takes several minutes to perform (**Table 1**).[9] Although most of what is seen is primary headache (tension and migraine), a careful examination of the CNs can be extremely valuable in elucidating important findings in secondary headaches and facial pain. These are often the patients who

---

Box 3
Ultraquick mental status examination

1. Orientation: name the month, day, year, and season

2. Attention and calculation: serial 7s

3. Memory: immediate recall of three objects (red ball, blue telephone, 66 Park Avenue); check recall of same three objects after 3 minutes

4. Speech: have patient name a watch and a body part (your wrist); have patient repeat the sentence "Today is a lovely day"; have patient follow a complex command (put your right hand on your left elbow)

Table 1
Clinical signs and symptoms of cranial nerves

Nerve	Function	Clinical Symptoms and Signs
Olfactory nerve (I)	Sensory	Anosmia or hyposmia
Optic nerve (II)	Sensory	Unilateral loss of visual acuity; may identify swollen disk; visual field loss (bitemporal hemianopia with lesions of the chiasm, lateral homonymous hemianopia with lesions of the optic tracts or optic radiations [often in quadrants])
Oculomotor nerve (III)	Motor and autonomic	Diplopia (vertical, horizontal, or oblique); ptosis; divergent strabismus; limited adduction; elevation and lowering of the eye; paralytic mydriasis (pupil 6–7 mm); accommodation paralysis
Trochlear nerve (IV)	Motor	Vertical diplopia looking down and to the healthy side, inclination and rotation of the head to the side opposite the lesion
Trigeminal nerve (V)	Mixed	Paresthesia or neuralgia of the hemiface, diminished corneal reflex, weakness of the muscles of mastication, drooping at the corners of the mouth
Abducens nerve (VI)	Motor	Horizontal diplopia, convergent strabismus, inability to abduct the eye
Facial nerve (VII)	Mixed	Peripheral facial paralysis (involving the forehead and the lower face) Loss of taste to the anterior two-thirds of the tongue, reduced lacrimal and salivary secretions
Acoustic nerve (VIII)	Sensory	Tinnitus (noises in the ear); hypoacusis or deafness (cochlear nerve) Vestibular syndrome (vestibular nerve)
Glossopharyngeal nerve (IX)	Mixed	Neuralgia, hypoesthesia, or anesthesia of the pharynx and posterior third of the tongue; loss of taste to the posterior tongue; paralysis of the velo-pharyngo-laryngeal junction; decreased salivary secretions
Vagus nerve (X)	Mixed	Hypoesthesia or anesthesia of the pharynx and larynx; paralysis of the velo-pharyngo-laryngeal junction; autonomic signs
Accessory nerve (XI)	Motor	Paralysis of sternocleidomastoid and trapezius muscles
Hypoglossal nerve (XII)	Motor	Paralysis of the hemitongue (deviation of the tongue to the affected side when protracted)

Data from Doyon et al. 2002; and *From* Barral JP, Croibier A. Pathologies of cranial nerves, manual therapy for the cranial nerves. Edinburgh (United Kingdom): Churchill Livingstone; 2009. p. 243–5.

have not responded to treatment despite visits to multiple specialists and emergency rooms. Their records (often electronic medical records) are voluminous and describe normal fundoscopic examinations, visual fields examinations, and detailed examinations of all the CNs and many other body parts. Be cautious. In many cases these are reimbursement-driven, computer-generated macros and the examinations described may not have been conducted at all.

Having worked with senior residents in family practice and internal medicine, I observe that most have essentially no confidence in their funduscopic examination or with their ability to conduct even a basic CN examination. These are bright, energetic young physicians who are often but months away from the daunting position of practicing either alone or with limited subspecialty backup in a remote town.

Key Points of the Examination

With the patient wearing their glasses or contact lenses, test visual acuity in each eye separately using a Snellen eye chart at 20 ft or Rosenbaum pocket card at 14 in. Examine the pupils for size and symmetry while checking for ptosis. Darken the room and gauge the pupil's reaction to light both direct (in the same eye) and consensual (in the other eye). The ophthalmoscope can be used as the light source.[10]

Inspect the optic disk for color, clarity of disk margins, and depth of the optic cup, and view all four quadrants of the retina checking for bleeding, exudates, vessel occlusion, and drusen (**Fig. 1**). If unable to adequately visualize the fundus for whatever reason, the examination is incomplete and this should be clearly noted in the medical records. Referral to an ophthalmologist is the logical next step.

Confrontation visual fields can be performed in each eye separately. These can reveal gross visual field deficits but are inadequate in establishing a baseline or in monitoring optic nerve function over time in such conditions as IIH pseudotumor cerebri (**Fig. 2**).

CN III, IV, and VI are tested by having the patient follow a finger with their eyes without moving their head. Test the six cardinal directions in an H pattern. Assess for failure of movement, nystagmus, convergence, and fatigability. In patients with facial pain the trigeminal nerve (CN V) sensory function can be tested with a sterile sharp item on the forehead, cheek, and jaw. The motor portion of CN V can be tested by having the patient open their mouth; clench their teeth (pterygoids); and by palpating the temporalis and masseter muscles as they clench. Inspecting facial symmetry, wrinkling the forehead, smiling, and shutting both the eyes tightly tests for the facial nerve (CN VII). I do not routinely test the corneal reflex.

On a selective basis the auditory nerve (CN VIII) can be crudely tested by using a tuning fork; CN IX and X (glossopharyngeal and vagus) by examining the palate for uvular displacement; and having the patients say "ah" and examining the symmetry

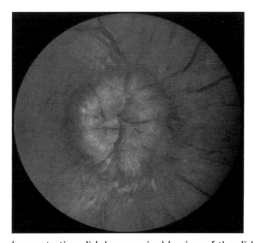

Fig. 1. Papilledema, demonstrating disk hyperemia, blurring of the disk borders, engorgement of the venules, and radial retinal folds at 6–7-o'clock (*Paton lines*). (*From* Osborne BJ, Liu GT, Newman NJ. Cranial nerve II and afferent visual pathways. In: Goetz CG, editor. Textbook of clinical neurology. 3rd edition. Philadelphia: W.B. Saunders; 2007. p. 113–32; and Sadun AA, Wang MY. Abnormalities of the optic disc. In: Kennard C, Leigh RJ, editors. Handbook of clinical neurology. vol. 102. Elsevier: 2011. p. 117–57.)

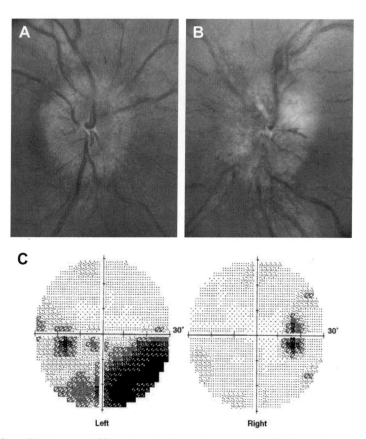

Fig. 2. Idiopathic intracranial hypertension (pseudotumor cerebri). The patient is a 39-year-old woman who had experienced brief episodes of vision loss in both eyes, lasting seconds, and headache. Magnetic resonance imaging findings were normal, and lumbar puncture revealed an opening pressure of 400 mm H_2O. Right eye (*A*) and left eye (*B*) show papilledema (bilateral optic disk swelling from elevated intracranial pressure). (*C*) Visual acuity was 20/20 in each eye, but visual field testing demonstrated enlargement of the blind spots bilaterally, and a visual field defect was evident in the left eye. This type of visual field defect ("nasal step") is characteristic of optic disk disease; it follows the nerve fiber layer pattern and respects the horizontal meridian. (*Data from* Palay DA, Krachmer JH, editors. Primary care ophthalmology. 2nd edition. Philadelphia: Mosby; 2005. p. 199–227.)

of the soft palate. The gag reflex (sensory CN IX, motor CN X) may be of interest when skull-base lesions are considered.

The accessory nerve (CN XI) supplies the sternocleidomastoid and trapezius muscles. The hypoglossal nerve (CN XII) is evaluated by listening to the clarity of the patient's speech, inspecting the tongue for wasting, fasiculations, and noting any asymmetry while protruding the tongue. The general rule is that the tongue deviates to the side of the pathology.

The rest of the examination including formal muscle strength testing and detailed sensory examination is not routinely performed and reserved for specialized situations in secondary headache, such as ischemic stroke and intraparenchymal and subdural hemorrhage where they may be of localizing value. It is always useful to watch the patient walk into the examining area and inspect their gait.

ANISOCORIA

Unilateral visual loss, even total blindness, does not result in anisocoria (**Box 4**).[11] Previous trauma and eye surgery, however, can result in differences in pupillary size. The swinging flashlight test is used to determine a relative afferent pupillary defect (**Fig. 3**). If there is pupillary dilatation in response to direct light stimulation (the consensual response is stronger than the direct response), this defines a relative afferent pupillary defect and suggests optic nerve dysfunction (optic neuropathy). In the middle panel in **Fig. 3**, there is considerable visual acuity loss in the left eye but both pupils are of equal size. In the right panel in **Fig. 3**, the left eye is affected by an optic neuropathy and a third nerve palsy. The pupils are unequal because of the oculoparasympathetic paresis associated with the left third nerve, and direct light stimulation of the left eye causes the right eye to dilate because of left optic neuropathy.

There are several important causes of unequal pupils to consider in headache evaluation. Essential anisocoria occurs in about 20% of the population.[12] The difference in pupillary size is 1 mm or less and there is no associated change in the reaction to light, movement of the eye, or ptosis (drooping of the lid). Horner's syndrome refers to symptoms caused by interruption of the lengthy sympathetic pathway from the brain to the eye including a central (first order), preganglionic (second order), and postganglionic (third order) segment (**Fig. 4**). The ptosis is less than 3 mm and ipsilateral to the pupil, which is rarely more than 2 mm smaller than the other side.[13] Facial anhydrosis is more commonly seen in acute lesions involving the first- and second-order neurons. The difference in pupillary size is more noticeable in dim light. In patients with headaches, Horner's syndrome is seen with carotid and vertebral dissection, Chiari 1 malformation, cluster, and with lung lesions and head and neck cancers (**Box 5**). Pharmacologic tests of the pupil are useful for localization and as a guide to direct imaging; however, in nonophthalmologic practices, these tests are rarely performed (**Fig. 5**). The key is recognition; Horner's syndrome in association with ipsilateral head or neck pain requires focused investigation for carotid or vertebral artery dissection.

Interruption of the sympathetic pathway results in a small pupil (Horner's syndrome). Parasympathetic preganglionic involvement associated with an oculomotor CN III nerve palsy presents with a large 6- to 7-mm dilated pupil (**Box 6**). Isolated mydriasis is not a manifestation of a CN III palsy, which is always accompanied by ptosis of greater degree than Horner's syndrome and impaired movement of the globe medially, upward and downward (**Fig. 6**). CN III palsy without pupillary involvement usually suggests microvascular ischemia (an infarct) rather than compression (an aneurysm) of CN III related to

---

Box 4
Characteristic pupillary abnormalities encountered in patients with or without headaches

1. Essential anisocoria (normal): 20% of population, 1–2 mm difference, remains unchanged in bright light and darkness, no associated ptosis

2. Tonic (Adie): the large pupil in bright light (may be smaller in darkness), absent response to light, sluggish response to near effort, with diminish deep tendon reflexes (DTRs) (Adie syndrome)

3. Horner's syndrome: small reactive pupil, ptosis, anhydrosis, iris may be lighter if congenital, more apparent in darkness

4. Oculomotor CN III nerve palsy: 6–7 mm dilated, fixed, more apparent in light, weak adduction, elevation and depression of the globe, eye droopy or shut

5. Pharmacologic: most dilated 9–10 mm, unreactive, does not constrict with 1% pilocarpine (CN III and Adie syndrome do constrict)

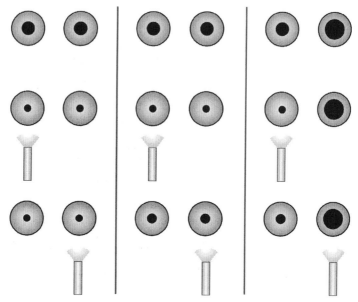

Fig. 3. Swinging flashlight test and the relative afferent pupillary defect. (*Left*) Normal swinging flashlight test, in which light directed in either eye elicits the same amount of pupillary constriction. (*Middle*) Swinging flashlight test revealing a left relative afferent pupillary defect in the hypothetical setting of visual loss in the left eye caused by an optic neuropathy. Pupillary sizes are equal at rest in ambient lighting. Light stimulation of the good right eye results in brisk bilateral pupillary constriction. Light stimulation of the visually impaired left eye produces comparatively weaker pupillary constriction, and both pupils dilate. (*Right*) Left third nerve palsy and optic neuropathy. The left pupil is fixed and dilated. When the light is shone into the good right eye, the right pupil constricts normally. When the light is shone into the left eye, however, the right pupil dilates because of the left optic neuropathy. (*Data from* Liu GT, Volpe NJ, Galetta SL. Neuro-opthalmology: diagnosis and management. 2nd edition. Philadelphia: W.B. Saunders Company; 2010.)

hypertension or diabetes.[14] A pupillary-sparing CN III that occurs in an individual younger than 50 without diabetes or vascular risk factors should undergo neuroimaging including computed tomography (CT) and computed tomographic angiography (CTA), or magnetic resonance imaging (MRI) and magnetic resonance angiography (MRA).

The pupillary-sparing CN III palsy associated with microvascular ischemia, diabetes, and hypertension is frequently painful but generally resolves spontaneously within 3 months (**Fig. 7**). An acute abducens CN VI nerve palsy can present in the context of the same vascular risk factors and improve spontaneously within a similar timeframe (**Box 7**). An acute third nerve palsy with pupillary involvement requires neuroimaging and is the result of a posterior communicating artery aneurysm until proved otherwise.[15] An acute third nerve palsy with pupillary sparing in a patient older than age 50 with the proper risk factors can be followed clinically without the need for emergent neuroimaging. I do perform laboratory studies including glucose, hemoglobin A_{1C}, erythrocyte sedimentation rate, and C-reactive protein. Giant cell arteritis can present in this age group as CN III palsy without pupillary involvement. If the third nerve palsy does not resolve within the anticipated 3 months, CT-CTA or MRI-MRA should be performed.

Adie tonic pupil can create a diagnostic challenge. It presents as painless anisocoria without paresis of the extraocular muscles. The tonic pupil is dilated and reacts poorly

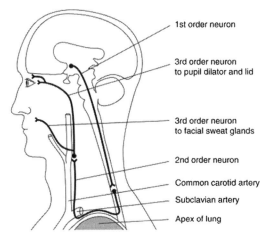

1st order neuron

3rd order neuron
to pupil dilator and lid

3rd order neuron
to facial sweat glands

2nd order neuron

Common carotid artery

Subclavian artery

Apex of lung

Fig. 4. Anatomy of sympathetic pathways to the eye. The sympathetic innervation of the eye consists of three neurons connected in series: first-order neurons, second-order neurons, and third-order neurons. The first-order neurons ("central" neurons) extend from the posterior hypothalamus to the C8-T2 level of the spinal cord. The second-order neurons ("preganglionic" neurons) leave the spinal cord and travel over the lung apex, around the subclavian artery, and along the carotid artery to the superior cervical ganglion. The third-order neurons ("postganglionic neurons") diverge and take two paths: those to the pupil and lid muscles travel along the internal carotid artery through the cavernous sinus to reach the orbit; those to the facial sweat glands travel with the external carotid artery to the face. Lesions in any of these neurons cause Horner's syndrome and distinct associated physical signs. (*Data from* McGee S, editor. Evidence-based physical diagnosis. 2nd edition. St Louis (MO): W.B. Saunders; 2007. p. 209–33.)

to light but better to near effort. It is more noticeable in bright light. The site of the lesion is believed to be postganglionic parasympathetic fibers in the ciliary ganglion or ciliary nerves within the orbit. It is usually not painful and other than recognition does not require neuroimaging studies. In individuals older than 50 presenting with a tonic pupil, I order erythrocyte sedimentation rate and C-reactive protein in that there is a rare but well-described association with giant cell (temporal) arteritis.[16]

Pharmacologic causes of the dilated pupil include installation (intentional or accidental) of any anticholinergic or sympathomimetic compound into the eye (dilating drops, contamination from scopolamine patches, jimson weed). Atropinized pupils are unusually large with diameters of 8 to 9 mm exceeding in size Adie tonic pupil or pupillary dilatation associated with CN III palsy.

Box 5
Causes of secondary headache associated with Horner's syndrome

1. First-order lesions: Chiari 1 malformation, basal skull tumors, brainstem infarction or hemorrhage, traumatic dissection of the vertebral artery

2. Second-order lesions: pulmonary apical lesions, subclavian artery aneurysm, apical lung tumor, mediastinal tumor, thyroid malignancies

3. Third-order lesions: cluster headache, internal carotid artery dissection, carotid cavernous fistula, cavernous sinus thrombosis, Tolosa-Hunt syndrome, giant cell arteritis

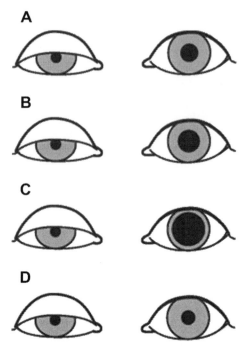

Fig. 5. Pupillary responses in Horner's syndrome (*A*) in light and (*B*) in dark. (*C*) After instillation of 10% cocaine the normal pupil dilates, the pupil that is sympathetically denervated shows no response regardless of location. (*D*) After instillation of 1% hydroxamphetamine, no response and the lesion is postganglionic (first- and second-order preganglionic lesions would have dilated). (*Data from* Schapira AH, editor. Neurology and clinical neuroscience. Philadelphia: Mosby; 2007. p. 260–73.)

Patients with unexplained anisocoria should undergo an ophthalmologic examination in that iritis, angle closure glaucoma, and prior eye surgery can all present with pupillary abnormalities. When presented with Horner's syndrome and ipsilateral headache or facial pain, consider carotid or vertebral dissection. When presented with a third nerve palsy with pupillary involvement, consider a posterior communicating artery aneurysm. When presented with third nerve palsy with pupillary sparing in an individual older than 50, consider diabetes or hypertension. When presented with a dilated tonic pupil that you correctly recognize as Adie pupil, consider yourself the DH, designated headache specialist.

Box 6
Headache conditions associated with oculomotor CN III palsy

1. Childhood migrainous ophthalmoplegia: migraine variant

2. Posterior communicating artery aneurysm: pupil dilated 7–8 mm

3. Diabetic ophthalmoplegia: pupil spared with third nerve muscles involved

4. Cavernous sinus thrombosis, Tolosa-Hunt syndrome, intracavernous aneurysm, mucormycosis, sphenoid sinusitis, mucocele or carcinoma, orbital pseudotumor, nasopharyngeal carcinoma, lymphoma

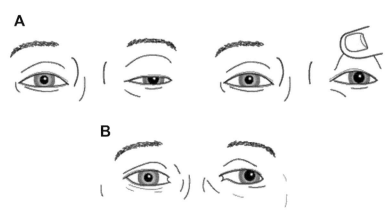

Fig. 6. (*A*) The patient with paresis of the left oculomotor nerve has typical findings: lateral deviation of the left eye, the left pupil dilated and unreactive to light, and the upper eyelid covering a portion of the pupil constituting ptosis. (*B*) In a milder case, close inspection reveals subtle ptosis, lateral deviation of the eye, and dilation of the pupil. In both cases, patients have diplopia that increases when looking to the right because this movement requires adducting the left eye; however, the paretic left medial rectus muscle cannot participate and the gaze becomes dysconjugate. (*Data from* Kaufman DM, editor. Clinical neurology for psychiatrists. 6th edition. Philadelphia: W.B. Saunders; 2007. p. 27–59.)

PAPILLEDEMA

Any physician or practitioner evaluating patients with headache should be competent in the funduscopic examination. As with any other skill, it is all about consistency, repetition, and experience. In my own practice, I have seen two patients with headaches who are now blind because of delayed treatment of IIH (pseudotumor cerebri). They had been evaluated in multiple emergency rooms, underwent several imaging studies both CT and MRI, were treated with a variety of medications, and reportedly had normal funduscopic examinations according to their electronic medical records but curiously do not remember those fundoscopic examinations even being conducted. One of medicine's dirtiest but poorly kept secrets in

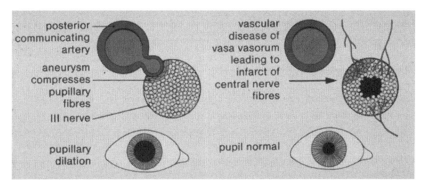

Fig. 7. Compressive lesions, such aneurysm and tumors (*left*), cause a complete CN 3 palsy, whereas microvascular lesions (*right*) spare the pupil. (*Data from* Able K, Shubrook J. A man with double vision, Osteopathic Family Physician. In: Slide Atlas of Ophthalmology. vol 2. Gower Medical Publishing; 2010. p. 175–9.)

Box 7
Headache conditions associated with abducens CN VI nerve palsy

1. Nonlocalizing: increased intracranial pressure, head trauma, post–lumbar puncture, spontaneous low CSF pressure or spinal anesthesia, diabetes or hypertension, or basal meningitis

2. Localizing:

    a. Cavernous sinus or superior orbital fissure (tumor, inflammation, aneurysm) often in combination with disorders of CN III and IV, and ophthalmic division of the trigeminal nerve CN V1; carotid-cavernous or dural arteriovenous fistula

    b. Clivus lesions: nasopharyngeal carcinoma or chordoma

    c. Cerebellopontine angle lesions (acoustic neuroma, meningioma); often in combination with disorders of CN VIII and VII, and first division of the trigeminal nerve V1

---

this age of computer-generated documents is that these very detailed physical examinations are more a representation of what should have happened rather than what actually did happen.

Papilledema refers to disk swelling exclusively caused by raised intracranial pressure. It is usually bilateral and central visual acuity is unaffected in contrast to other conditions with swollen disks (**Fig. 8**). The subarachnoid space of the brain is continuous with the optic nerve sheath and, as CSF pressure increases, its transmission into the sheath impedes axoplasmic flow. When one looks at the optic nerve with an ophthalmoscope one is actually viewing the buildup of this axoplasmic material resulting in the characteristic swelling at the nerve head (see **Fig. 1**).

Funduscopic findings in the early stage include disk hyperemia, small hemorrhages in the nerve fiber layer, and obliteration of spontaneous venous pulsations when the CSF pressure exceeds 200 mm H_2O. Spontaneous venous pulsations are present normally in 80% of the population.[17] Their absence is not diagnostic but their presence is useful in excluding papilledema. An abducens CN VI palsy may be present as a nonlocalizing sign of increased intracranial pressure (**Fig. 9**). As the process worsens the vessels at the disk margins become blurred, the disk becomes elevated at its borders and in distinct.[18] The peripapillary retina develops concentric or radial folds (Paton lines) (see **Fig. 1**).

If papilledema persists for months, the disk hyperemia and swelling eventually subside giving way to a pale atrophic disk that has lost its central cup. In the early phase, visual fields may be normal.[19] As the process worsens, the disk enlarges as does the physiologic blind spot. Eventually nerve fibers are destroyed resulting in severely constricted fields, optic atrophy, and ultimately loss of central visual acuity. The goal is to recognize the process in the early stages, institute aggressive treatment, and prevent visual loss.

Fundoscopy of the swollen disk is all about pattern recognition but it has been estimated that less than 10% of physicians feel proficient in direct ophthalmoscopic evaluation of the fundus (**Table 2**).[20] There is hope in technologic innovation, such as nonmydriatic funduscopic cameras. These can be operated by nurses or other technical personnel and images of the fundus can be stored and evaluated either by a computer or a specialist in ophthalmology (**Fig. 10**).

A conservative estimate suggests that in more than 80% of patients with headaches the funduscopic evaluation is either inadequate or omitted entirely.[21] These devices are still evolving but, in the face of widespread, inadequate availability of accurate fundoscopy, they make sense and it is hoped they will find their way at the least into the emergency room.[22] CT and MRI revolutionized evaluation of the brain and spine, and

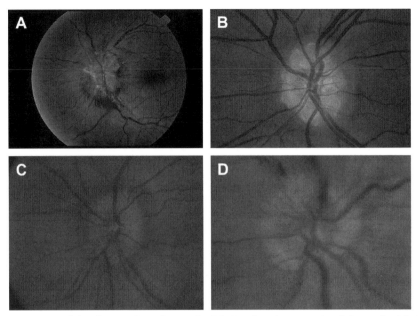

Fig. 8. Images of the abnormal swollen optic disk. Fundus photographs of the optic disk. (*A*) Acute papilledema with disk swelling, exudates, and hemorrhages. (*B*) Pseudopapilledema with optic nerve head drusen. (*C*) Acute optic neuritis with mild disk edema without hemorrhages. (*D*) Acute anterior ischemic optic neuropathy disk swelling with hemorrhages seen superiorly. Can be seen in giant cell (temporal) arteritis. (*Data from* Graves JS, Galetta SL. Acute visual loss and other neuro-ophthalmologic emergencies: management. Neurol Clin 2012;30(1):75–99.)

practicing without them seems unimaginable. The optic nerve and retina await a similar technologic advance. In the real world of primary care headache management, there is a growing void between the clinical advances and patient access to their benefits. This has been accentuated by shortages in manpower.

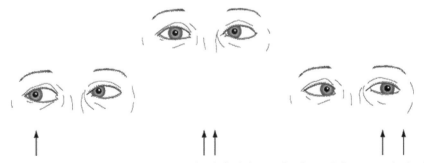

Fig. 9. In the center picture, a patient with a left abducens (sixth cranial) nerve palsy looks straight ahead. The patient's left eye is deviated medially. The eyes are dysconjugate, and the patient sees two *arrows* when looking ahead. In the picture on the left, the patient looks to the right. The eyes are conjugate, and the patient sees only a single *arrow*. In the picture on the right, the patient looks to the left. The paretic left eye fails to cross the midline laterally, it fails to abduct. The exaggeration of the dysconjugate gaze increases the diplopia. (*Data from* Visual disturbances. In: Kaufman DM, editor. Clinical neurology for psychiatrists. 6th edition. Philadelphia: W.B. Saunders; 2007. p. 267–94.)

Table 2
Differential diagnosis of the abnormal swollen optic disk

Cause	History	Fundoscopic Appearance	Visual Examination	Ancillary Diagnostic Tests
Increased intracranial pressure (papilledema)	Morning headache, transient visual obscurations, double vision, tinnitus, nausea	Usually bilateral; disk hyperemia, cup preserved (early), cotton wool spots, exudates, obscuration of retinal vessels, absence of spontaneous venous pulsations	No APD, central acuity spared, no color loss, enlarged blind spot, visual field constriction, and inferior nasal defect	MRI/MRV of head; lumbar puncture (document opening pressure, rule out infection)
Drusen pseudopapilledema	Usually asymptomatic	Glistening hyaline bodies, absence of disk hyperemia, hemorrhage, or exudate; anomalous retinal vessels with central origination and trifurcations, irregular disk border, absent cup	Normal examination or irregular peripheral field constriction, enlarged blind spot; normal visual acuity	CT or orbital ultrasound may visualize calcified hyaline bodies
Optic neuritis	History of multiple sclerosis (or other inflammatory disorder); retro-orbital pain on eye movement, if demyelinating may worsen with heat (Uhthoff phenomenon)	Variable disk swelling, typically mild (retrobulbar involvement has normal disk appearance); usually unilateral in adults	APD; loss of central acuity and color discrimination; central or centrocecal scotoma	MRI for evidence of demyelination; CSF for pleocytosis and oligoclonal bands, IgG index and synthesis rate
Ischemia (anterior ischemic optic neuropathy)	Sudden painless loss of vision; >50 y of age; hypertension, diabetes, history of hypotensive episode	Usually unilateral; segmental disk edema; other eye may show absent cup	Variable field abnormality; often altitudinal; acuity variably affected; APD common	Work-up for hypertension, diabetes, vasculitis, giant cell arteritis (glucose, BP, erythrocyte sedimentation rate, C-reactive protein)
Infection	History of known infection or compromised immune status; systemic symptoms, such as fever, meningismus, other focal neurologic deficits	May be bilateral or asymmetric disk swelling with or without exudates, may also be associated with a macular star		Head CT or MRI, infectious work-up, including serologic and CSF studies (HIV, Lyme disease, cat-scratch disease, and other as appropriate)
Infiltrative	History of neoplasm, sarcoid, or other infiltrative disease; focal eye pain	Possible disk elevation and swelling; pallor	Variable field abnormality and acuity loss	MRI of the brain and orbits; CSF for pleocytosis and cytology

Abbreviation: APD, Afferent pupillary defect.

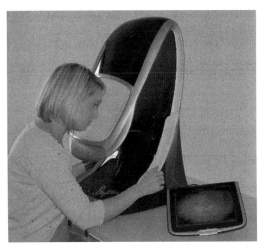

Fig. 10. Nonmydriatic fundus photography. (*Courtesy of* Optos, NA; Marlborough, MA; with permission.)

Evaluation of CN V and VII is simple and very important in the evaluation of facial pain.[23] The trigeminal nerve CN V supplies the masseter muscle and the lateral pterygoid muscle, sensation to the upper face V1, mid-face V2, and lower face V3. Lesions of the trigeminal nerve cause difficulty clenching the jaw (masseter) and moving it from side to side (lateral pterygoid). Diminished sensation of the face is of localizing value.

The numb chin syndrome involving diminished sensation of the lower lip and chin has been identified as a potential sign of metastatic involvement in either the mandible or skull base. In trigeminal neuralgia the function of CN V is normal and any abnormal findings should prompt evaluation into secondary causes (**Box 8**).[24] Although the trigeminal nerve serves as the afferent limb of the corneal reflex, I have found this reflex to be of limited clinical value and uncomfortable; I no longer test it.

Lesions of the facial nerve cause weakness of the muscles of facial expression including smiling, wrinkling the forehead, eyelid closure, and blinking. There may be problems identified with tearing, hyperacusis, and taste on the anterior two-thirds of the tongue. Peripheral lesions of CN VII involve the upper and lower facial muscles. Central lesions involving the contralateral motor cortex and pyrimidal tract generally spare the forehead.

Simultaneous involvement of CN V and VII should alert to the possibility of perineural tumor spread or growth of neoplasm, frequently malignant, along the nerve trunk

---

Box 8
Clinical points regarding CN V, the trigeminal nerve, and CN VII, the facial nerve

1. Trigeminal neuralgia implies normal motor and sensory function of the trigeminal nerve.

2. Other than pain behind the ear at the very onset, Bell's palsy is not a painful condition.

3. Bell palsy is but one cause of a peripheral CN VII palsy and is a diagnosis of exclusion.

4. Atypical facial pain is not a diagnosis but rather the lack of one.

5. The combination of objective trigeminal sensory loss and facial weakness constitutes a red flag for an underlying head and neck malignancy and possible perineural tumor spread.

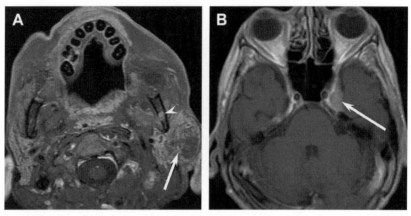

Fig. 11. Magnetic resonance image for perineural spread. (*A*) Axial contrast-enhanced T1-weighted image shows a large enhancing left parotid mass (*arrow*) with abnormal enhancement in the mandibular foramen (*arrowhead*) related to perineural spread along the auriculotemporal nerve to the mandibular nerve. (*B*) More superior image reveals abnormal enhancement in left Meckel cave (*arrow*) from perineural spread of the parotid tumor intracranially. (*Data from* Gluck I, Ibrahim M, Popovtzer A, et al. Skin cancer of the head and neck with perineural invasion: defining the clinical target volumes based on the pattern of failure. Int J Radiat Oncol Biol Phys 2009;74(1):38–46.)

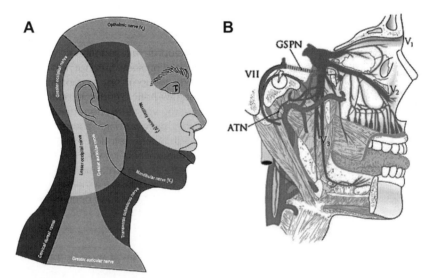

Fig. 12. Major nerves innervating facial skin and musculature. (*A*) Facial skin regions according to distribution of the various sensory nerves (note that skin tumors at any facial site can spread by the respective sensory nerve and by cranial nerve VII if the underlying muscle is invaded by tumor). (*B*) CN V and VII and their connections (note the auriculotemporal nerve [ATN] and greater superficial petrosal nerve [GSPN] connecting CN VII with V3 and V2, respectively, allowing tumor spread between these nerves). (*Data from* Gluck I, Ibrahim M, Popovtzer A, et al. Skin cancer of the head and neck with perineural invasion: defining the clinical target volumes based on the pattern of failure. Int J Radiat Oncol Biol Phys 2009;74(1):38–46.)

(**Fig. 11**).[25] Head and neck cancers including squamous cell carcinoma, adenoid cystic carcinoma of the parotid, and lymphoma are the most common neoplasms that exhibit this behavior.[26,27] Be wary of the patient with facial pain and facial weakness and be hesitant in attributing the facial weakness to an old CN VII palsy (Bell's). There are numerous anatomic connections between these CNs (**Fig. 12**) and this condition is frequently not recognized or mistakenly attributed to Bell's palsy or trigeminal neuralgia with significant medical and medicolegal consequences (see **Box 8**).

SUMMARY

The population of patients suffering with headaches is vast and underserved. The most critical element in headache evaluation is the history. The targeted history not only differentiates primary from secondary headaches but also provides a realistic list of conditions associated with secondary headache. Several of these conditions do present with specific physical findings, such as papilledema, Horner's syndrome, or CN palsy. The targeted physical examination of the patient with headache takes less than 3 minutes. The ability simply to recognize but a few straightforward clinical findings directs the evaluation in the proper direction. If you enjoy seeing patients, feel competent identifying but a few physical findings, and understand the basics of primary and secondary headaches and facial pain, there is urgent need of your services.

REFERENCES

1. Hazard E, Munakata J, Bigal ME, et al. The burden of migraine in the United States: current and emerging perspectives on disease management and economic analysis. Value Health 2009;12(1):55–64.
2. Rothner AD. Complicated migraine and migraine variants. Semin Pediatr Neurol 2001;8(1):7–12.
3. Morgan R, King D, Clerkin L. Fundus12. Copy: a forgotten art? Postgrad Med J 1999;75:282–4.
4. International Headache Society Classification Subcommittee. The international classification of headache disorders, 2nd edition. Cephalalgia 2004;24(Suppl 1): 1–151.
5. Tronvik E, Stovner LJ, Hagen K, et al. High pulse pressure protects against headache: prospective and cross-sectional data (HUNT study). Neurology 2008;70: 1329–36.
6. Hagen K, Stovner LJ, Vatten L, et al. Blood pressure and risk of headache: a prospective study of 22,685 adults in Norway. J Neurol Neurosurg Psychiatry 2002;72:463–6.
7. Gu Q, Dillon CF, Burt VL, et al. Association of hypertension treatment and control with all-cause and cardiovascular disease mortality among US adults with hypertension. Am J Hypertens 2010;23:38–45.
8. Al-Twaijri WA, Shevell MI. Pediatric migraine equivalents: occurrence and clinical features in practice. Pediatr Neurol 2002;26:365–8.
9. DeMyer WE. Technique of the neurological examination. 5th edition. New York: McGraw-Hill Professional; 2003.
10. Bates B. Nervous system. In: A guide to physical examination and history taking. 10th edition. Philadelphia: Lippincott, Williams & Wilkins; 2008. p. 497–573.
11. Wilhelm H. Disorders of the pupil. In: Christopher Kennard, R. John Leigh, editors. Handbook of clinical neurology. vol. 102. 2011. p. 427–66.

12. Lam BL, Thompson HS, Corbett JJ. The prevalence of simple anisocoria. Am J Oph-thalmol 1987;104:69–73.

13. Almog Y, Gepstein R, Kessler A. Diagnostic value of imaging in Horner syndrome in adults. J Neuroophthalmol 2010;30:7–11.

14. Miller NR, Newman NJ, et al, editors. Walsh & Hoyt's clinical neuro-ophthalmology: the essentials. 2nd edition. Philadelphia: Lippincott Williams & Wilkins; 2008. p. 122–45.

15. Brazis PW. Isolated palsies of cranial nerves III, IV, and VI. Semin Neurol 2009; 29(1):14–28.

16. Faroozan R, Buono L, Savino P, et al. Tonic pupils from giant cell arteritis. Br J Ophthalmol 2003;87(4):510–2.

17. Sadun A, Wang M. Abnormalities of the optic disc. In: Kennard C, Leigh R, editors. Handbook of clinical neurology. vol. 102. 2011. p. 117–57.

18. Ehlers JP, Shah CP. Papilledema. In: The Wills Eye Manual: Office and Emer-gency Room Diagnosis and Treatment of Eye Disease. 5th edition. Baltimore, MD: Lippincott Williams & Wilkins; 2008. p. 252–4.

19. Vaphiades MS. The disk edema dilemma. Surv Ophthalmol 2002;47(2):183–8.

20. Friedman DI, Jacobson DM. Diagnostic criteria for idiopathic intracranial hyper-tension [abstract]. Neurology 2002;59:1492–5.

21. Cahill V, Willetts E, Nicholl D, et al. The TOS study: can we improve the ophthal-mological assessment of medical patients by foundation year doctors?. Abstracts from the Association of British Neurologists Annual Meeting 2011. J Neurol Neu-rosurg Psychiatry 2012;83:e1. http://dx.doi.org/10.1136/jnnp-2011-301993.78.

22. Cozma I, Fraser S, Nambiar AK, et al. How to use an ophthalmoscope. Career Focus. [Online]. BMJ 2004;329(7461):55–6. Available at: http://careers.bmj.com/careers/advice/view-article.html?id=354. Accessed December 30, 2011.

23. Bruce B, Lamirel C, Biousse V, et al. Feasibility of nonmydriatic ocular fundus photography in the emergency department: phase I of the FOTO-ED study. Acad Emerg Med 2011;18(9):928–33.

24. Macleod J, Douglas G, Nicol F, et al. Macleod's clinical examination. 12th edition. Edinburgh (United Kingdom): Churchhill Livingstone Elsevier; 2009.

25. Gronseth G, Cruccu G, Alksne J, et al. Practice parameter: the diagnostic evaluation and treatment of trigeminal neuralgia (an evidence-based review): report of the Quality Standards Subcommittee of the American Academy of Neurology and the European Federation of Neurological Societies. Neurology 2008;71(15):1183–90.

26. Lee C, Watson RE, Given CA. Evaluation of retrograde tumor spread via pterygo-maxillary fissure and trigeminal nerve [paper]. Am J Roentgenol 2000;174(3):18.

27. Mendenhall WM, Amdur RJ, Hinerman RW, et al. Skin cancer of the head and neck with perineural invasion. Am J Clin Oncol 2007;30(1):93–6.

The Role of Laboratory Testing in the Evaluation of Headache

Charles D. Donohoe, MD

KEYWORDS

- Secondary headache • Targeted laboratory studies • False-positives
- High-risk or special situations • CSF studies

KEY POINTS

- Laboratory tests play a diagnostic role in a few select secondary headaches and are not useful in primary headache disorders.
- Tests should be ordered based on specific clues derived from the history and clinical examination.
- A shotgun approach to testing that includes diseases of low prevalence often yields false-positive results and resultant misdiagnosis.
- Cerebrospinal fluid analysis can be important in secondary headache evaluation but is often delayed or omitted.

INTRODUCTION

Testing blood and urine has a minor role in the evaluation of headaches. Most headaches represent a benign primary disorder, most often migraine or tension-type headache, that are identified based on diagnostic criteria obtained from the history. In general, further diagnostic tests including imaging (computed tomography [CT] and magnetic resonance imaging [MRI]), and blood and urine tests are unnecessary. Electroencephalography (EEG) and plain radiographs of the skull no longer have any primary role in headache evaluation.

Unnecessary testing is expensive and has risks, particularly when dealing with conditions with low prevalence. Many of the results are incidental to the patient's symptoms and represent statistical false-positives. Further diagnostic studies and treatments based on these false-positives can result in morbidity and even mortality.

This article highlights the limited number of conditions in which blood work plays a major role in headache diagnosis.

Testing is reserved for secondary headaches, which are found in patients who do not neatly fit diagnostic criteria and have not responded to therapy.

Department of Neurology, University of Missouri Kansas City School of Medicine, 17020 E.40Hwy. Suite 8, Independence, MO 64055, USA
E-mail address: charles.d.donohoe@gmail.com

Med Clin N Am 97 (2013) 217–224
http://dx.doi.org/10.1016/j.mcna.2012.12.002
0025-7125/13/$ – see front matter © 2013 Elsevier Inc. All rights reserved.

These patients may present acutely or may be chronically ill and display red flags (**Box 1**). Many patients have searched the Internet on their own. These patients have an acute explosive headache or a chronic debilitating headache. Some of these frustrated, almost desperate patients have been seen by multiple physicians in different specialties but remain without either an effective therapy or a diagnosis that makes sense. They usually have had brain CT or MRI or both. They often have had extensive blood work on multiple occasions. What they are lacking is a physician willing to spend the time to obtain a thorough, targeted history that probes for the various conditions (listed in **Table 1**) that are frequently subject to misdiagnosis or delayed diagnosis, a personal review of their neuroimaging studies, a brief neurologic examination including examination of their optic fundi, and often spinal fluid analysis. This article includes the role of cerebrospinal fluid (CSF) laboratory analysis in headache evaluation.

WHAT TESTS SHOULD I ORDER?

This is the most important question, and it can only be answered by considering 2 other questions: what am I looking for, and how will this change my management of the patient with headache? This approach applies to blood work (**Box 2**), CSF analysis (**Box 3**) and neuroimaging (CT and MRI). The answers are a function of the data derived from the history and, less so, from the physical examination. It is mainly the history that formulates the list of reasonable diagnostic possibilities and guides the proper selection of diagnostic tests. Spending more time on the history avoids wasting your patient's money on unnecessary tests.

As you review the list of important conditions (see **Table 1**), blood work is an essential component in only few, including meningitis (complete blood count [CBC], blood cultures), temporal arteritis (erythrocyte sedimentation rate [ESR], C-reactive protein [CRP]), headache associated with hypothyroidism (thyroid-stimulating hormone [TSH], thyroxin [T4]), and carbon monoxide intoxication (CO, carboxyhemoglobin level).

Testing for diseases of low prevalence in a particular area generally yields more false-positives than true-positives. This situation can be improved by reserving testing for those with historical or physical findings specific to the disease. Lyme disease is an example of a disease with low prevalence in most of the United States and testing should be reserved for those with distinct findings such as erythema migrans or Bell's

---

Box 1
Red flags in headache diagnosis

- A new headache in an individual older than 40 years or a group of severe headaches that begin suddenly (thunderclap headaches)
- The worst headache of a patient's life or headaches in an individual with a family history of cerebral aneurysm
- Headaches associated with fever, encephalopathy, stiff neck, or rash, or following head injury, during pregnancy, and post partum headaches
- Headache in an individual immunologically compromised (cancer, human immunodeficiency virus [HIV])
- Headaches associated with exercise, sexual intercourse, coughing, weight lifting, and Valsalva
- Headaches associated with focal findings such as aphasia, ataxia, hemiparesis, papilledema, or oculomotor disturbance

Table 1
Important causes of secondary headache

Causes	Appropriate Tests
Hemorrhage (subarachnoid, epidural, subdural, intraparenchymal, pituitary)	CT/MRI
Meningitis	CSF, CBC, blood cultures
Encephalitis	MRI, CSF
Chiari 1 malformation	MRI
Hydrocephalus	MRI
Neoplasm	MRI
Venous sinus thrombosis	MRI/MRV
Sphenoid sinusitis	MRI
Carotid/vertebral dissection	MRI/MRA
Idiopathic intracranial hypertension	CSF
Low CSF pressure headache spontaneous/after lumbar puncture	MRI
Temporal (giant cell) arteritis	ESR, CRP, biopsy temporal artery
Carbon monoxide intoxication	Carboxyhemoglobin, CO level
Open-angle glaucoma	Ophthalmologic examination
Headache associated with hypothyroidism	TSH, T4

Abbreviations: CBC, complete blood count; CRP, C-reactive protein; CSF, cerebrospinal fluid; ESR, erythrocyte sedimentation rate; MRA, magnetic resonance angiography; MRV, magnetic resonance venography; TSH, thyroid-stimulating hormone; T4, thyroxin.

Box 2
Useful blood tests in the evaluation of secondary headache

Basic panel:

   CBC: infection, malignancy, giant cell arteritis

   ESR, CRP: giant cell arteritis

   Chemical profile

   Blood cultures: meningitis

   Protime, prothrombin time INR (International Normalized Ratio) (for patients on coumadin anticoagulation). PTT, partial thromboplastin time (for patients on heparin).

   TSH: about 30% of patients with hypothyroidism have headaches that generally resolve within 2 months after effective treatment

   Because of high false-positive rates, I avoid routine use of Lyme (enzyme-linked immunosorbent assay) test, Antinuclear Antibody Test (ANA), Venereal Disease Laboratory Test (VDRL) unless there are strong supporting clinical features that suggest the disease

High-risk situations

   HIV, hepatitis C, carboxyhemoglobin: the CDC recommends HIV testing for everyone aged 13 to 64 years, and testing for hepatitis C for all baby boomers born between 1945 and 1966

Rare genetic conditions associated with headache:

   CADISIL: NOTCH3 mutations on chromosome 19

   MELAS: mitochondrial DNA

> **Box 3**
> **CSF analysis in headache evaluation**
>
> Abnormal CSF opening pressure of more than 250 mm H_2O: must be measured in the lateral recumbent position with legs extended
>
> Tube 1 (2 mL): cell count
>
> There should be 0 RBCs, fewer than 5 lymphocytes, and 0 polymorphonuclear leukocytes. Traumatic taps occur in 10% to 30%. One additional WBC is allowed for each 700 RBCs.
>
> Tube 2 (2 mL): Gram stain, culture, and sensitivity including fungi and mycobacterium
>
> In situations in which meningitis is suspected, I order reverse transcriptase enterovirus polymerase chain reaction (PCR), broad-based bacterial PCR, and herpes simplex virus (HSV)-1 and HSV-2 PCR.
>
> In immunocompromised patients, add varicella-zoster PCR, cryptococcal antigen, India ink prep, tuberculosis PCR, histoplasma antigen, PCR for cytomegalovirus DNA, interleukin-10 for primary central nervous system lymphoma, JC viral PCR for progressive multifocal leukoencephalopathy, and VDRL (syphilis).
>
> Tube 3 (2 mL): protein (15–60 mg/dL) and glucose (40–80 mg/dL)
>
> Tube 4 (2 mL): cell count for comparison with tube 1, particularly if concerned about traumatic tap
>
> RBC counts in tube 4 less than 500/mm^3 or a 70% reduction in RBC count from tube 1 to Tube 4 suggest a traumatic tap rather than subarachnoid hemorrhage.[a]
>
> [a] If CSF glucose is 70% lower than serum glucose, suspect bacterial infection or carcinomatous meningitis. CSF protein is increased by about 1 mg/dL for every 750 RBCs.

palsy. Misdiagnosis based on unvalidated laboratory tests is common, with serious individual and public health consequences. The controversial entity of a chronic Lyme disease state is an evolving example of the tenuous relationship between science, clinical medicine, patient advocacy, and politics.

SPECIAL SITUATIONS

Hypothyroidism is a common disorder and about 30% of patients with hypothyroidism complain of headache. The combination of an increased TSH level and low T4 supports the diagnosis of primary hypothyroidism. Effective treatment may be associated with headache improvement within 2 months.

Carbon monoxide (CO) is a leading cause of intentional and unintentional poisoning. The most common symptom associated with this colorless, odorless toxin is headache followed by dizziness and nausea. Misdiagnosis as migraine is a common error. Exposure is often associated with faulty heating and vehicle exhaust systems. Although the diagnosis is often considered when several individuals who share the same residence present with similar symptoms, misdiagnosis or delayed diagnosis is common, with tragic consequences. The cognitive and neuropsychiatric symptoms seen with chronic CO exposure are particularly prone to diagnostic error.

Normal individuals in urban areas may have CO levels as high as 5%. Smokers may have chronically increased CO levels of as high as 10%. As the CO level increases acutely from 10% to 40%, headaches become more severe, as does the associated nausea, disequilibrium, and vomiting. Levels of more than 40% to 50% result in impaired consciousness and death. The half-life of CO is about 5 hours, so prompt measurement following suspected exposure is critical.

Unrelated to headache evaluation, the US Centers for Disease Control and Prevention (CDC) has recommended HIV testing for all individuals ages 13 to 64 years and hepatitis C testing for all individuals born between 1946 and 1966. There are now more deaths in the United States associated with hepatitis C than HIV. We have observed a tendency for physicians and patients to ignore these important recommendations, often because of nothing more than a visceral sense of social awkwardness.

Cerebral autosomal dominant arteriopathy with subcortical infarcts and leukoencephalopathy (CADISIL) is a genetic disorder that affects small blood vessels in the brain with attacks of migraine with aura and the MRI findings of multiple confluent white matter lesions often localized to the anterior temporal lobes or external capsule. These patients often have close relatives who have experienced stroke at an early age. Diagnostic confirmation consists of either skin biopsy or blood testing for NOTCH3 mutations on chromosome 19. This testing involves DNA sequencing and is expensive, technically difficult, and belongs within the province of the headache specialist.

Mitochondrial encephalopathy, lactic acidosis, and strokelike episodes (MELAS) is a complicated multisystem disease associated with point or microdeletion mutations in mitochondrial DNA. Migraine, strokelike episodes, seizures, and psychiatric symptoms are common. The disease may initially present in a benign fashion as migraine but eventually becomes more complex, including seizures, cardiomyopathy, and resultant stroke. Death often occurs before age 40 years.

Maternally derived mitochondrial DNA is 10 times more prone to mutation than somatic DNA. Blood tests may show increased levels of lactate and pyruvate but diagnostic confirmation requires mitochondrial DNA analysis, which is now commercially available. DNA obtained from muscle biopsies or hair follicles may be more reliable than testing leukocytes. As with CADISIL, this specialized and expensive testing is not routinely ordered.

Temporal (Giant Cell) Arteritis

Temporal arteritis is the most common form of systemic vasculitis and adults and is one of the few headache conditions in which laboratory tests play a role. Headache in any location is the most prominent symptom and is not necessarily confined to the temporal region or associated with tender, cordlike temporal arteries. This disease most often affects white women more than 50 years of age of northern European descent. Smoking is an additional risk factor.

More significant than the location of the headache and the presence of second temporal arteries are the associated symptoms of malaise, fatigue, scalp tenderness, jaw claudication, and polymyalgia rheumatica. The proximal shoulder girdle can have pain, and weakness associated with polymyalgia rheumatica may develop before or after the signs of temporal arteritis.

Visual disturbances including blurred vision, amaurosis fugax, and scintillations caused by retinal ischemia may cause further diagnostic confusion with primary headache conditions such as migraine with aura. The major complication of temporal arteritis is visual loss caused by retinal ischemia and the condition should be approached as an ophthalmologic emergency.

Any patient with a strong clinical history is at risk for visual loss and treatment with steroids should not be delayed. Pretreatment with steroids does not affect the results of temporal artery biopsy and positive biopsies have been reported even 6 months after the institution of corticosteroids.

Temporal arteritis is an inflammatory process and is associated with the increase of acute phase reactants. I order a CBC, ESR, CRP, and complete chemical profile.

Findings often include a microcytic anemia and thrombocytosis. Several studies suggest that a platelet count greater than 375,000 per µL is more sensitive than an increased ESR or CRP in identifying temporal arteritis. Alkaline phosphatase is also frequently increased in 20% to 30% of cases.

The ESR usually ranges from 60 to 110 mm/hour in temporal arteritis. However, it can be normal in up to 20% of biopsy-proven cases. The ESR increases with age. For women, the general rule is age plus 10/2, for men it is age/2. I order both ESR and CRP. CRP is not affected by age. Although they are both usually increased, it is common to find discordant results. In my experience, this most commonly consists of a normal ESR but an increased CRP.

Laboratory studies such as ESR, CRP, and platelet count support the clinical impression but their absence, and even a negative temporal artery biopsy, does not rule it out. Increasing the length of the temporal artery removed during biopsy to 2.5 cm increases the diagnostic yield, but false-negatives still exist. The major impact of missing or delaying this diagnosis is significant visual loss associated with the arteritic variant of anterior ischemic optic neuropathy, which can be bilateral. Treatment is long-term and even lifetime treatment with steroids. Faced with such prolonged therapy with an agent with serious side effects, a positive biopsy is reassuring for both the patient and the physician. Some specialists even recommend the initial approach of bilateral temporal artery biopsies but, in clinical practice, this is generally not the standard.

It is most important to work with a surgeon and pathologist experienced in the nuances of this disease who are dedicated to the proper surgical processing and histologic evaluation of this tissue. This combination may not be readily accessible and it is often best to consider referral to a center with more experience.

Urine Drug Screening

Patients with both primary and secondary headaches are frequently evaluated in emergency rooms where the index of suspicion for drug-seeking behavior and toxicity remains understandably high. This climate fosters the frequent implementation of urine drug screening (UDS) into the evaluation algorithm, often without a clear rationale. These preliminary drug-screening tests performed by immunoassay have multiple technical limitations including numerous false-positive results associated with many frequently prescribed and over-the-counter medications. The understanding of the limitations of UDS and the necessity for confirmation of unexplained positive results with gas chromatography–mass spectrometry is essential in avoiding medical error and unjust damage to the patient's reputation. In the face of this complexity and additional expense without defined benefit, we discourage the routine use of UDS in headache management.

Lumbar Puncture and CSF Analysis

Unlike blood work, lumbar puncture and CSF analysis is more often a critical component in the evaluation of secondary headaches. However, because lumbar puncture is perceived as cumbersome, it is frequently neglected, often resulting in delay or misdiagnosis. This point is subject to some debate but we recommend that lumbar puncture in headache evaluation be performed after brain neuroimaging, either CT or MRI. Although the risk of brain herniation secondary to an unsuspected intracranial mass is extremely small, it is indefensible.

Measurement of CSF pressure is critical in the diagnosis of idiopathic intracranial hypertension (pseudotumor cerebri). It requires that the measurement be performed in the lateral recumbent position with the legs extended. CSF cannot be properly measured with patients either prone (lying on their stomachs, as frequently was the case when performed by radiologists under fluoroscopy) or sitting upright. The upper limit of CSF pressure considered to be normal is 250 mm of water.

Subarachnoid hemorrhage most commonly associated with aneurysmal rupture is a particularly treacherous cause of secondary headache, with inherently high morbidity, mortality, and an initial misdiagnosis rate of 25%. Roughly two-thirds of untreated patients either die or have significant neurologic disability. A noncontrast CT brain is 95% sensitive in identifying subarachnoid blood during the first 24 hours following the initial ictus, but this decreases to 50% within a week. Patients seen several days after the onset, or patients whose CT results are equivocal, should undergo lumbar puncture.

CSF pressure should always be measured, and high pressures provide an important clue regarding cerebral venous sinus thrombosis and pseudotumor cerebri. The presence of red cells in the spinal fluid is diagnostic for subarachnoid hemorrhage. However, 10% to 30% of lumbar punctures are traumatic. From 4% to 6% of the population has an incidental intracranial aneurysm, which further complicates the misinterpretation of a traumatic lumbar puncture exposing the patient to unnecessary and potentially risky diagnostic and therapeutic interventions.

The differentiation of a traumatic tap from subarachnoid hemorrhage is not clear-cut. The time-honored method of identifying diminished erythrocyte count in successive tubes is not reliable. Spinning down the CSF and examining the supernatant for xanthochromia also has limitations. Hemoglobin is metabolized to oxyhemoglobin, a reddish pink pigment, generally within 2 to 3 hours following the ictus. The formation of bilirubin resulting in the yellow xanthochromic color requires an enzyme-dependent process that requires up to 12 hours to occur. Its appearance is more reliable when identified by spectrophotometry rather than the naked eye. However, spectrophotometry is not always available. In subarachnoid hemorrhage, xanthochromia identified by spectrophotometry is usually present within 12 hours and persists for 2 weeks.

CSF red blood cell (RBC) counts of more than 10,000 per mm^3 usually indicate subarachnoid hemorrhage. Cell counts less than 500 per mm^3 coupled with a decrease of 70% in RBCs from tube #1 to 4 indicate a traumatic tap. Patients in whom the history and clinical setting are strongly suspicious should undergo CT angiography (CTA) or magnetic resonance angiography (MRA), both of which have become more technically accurate and clinically available.

In the evaluation of secondary headache associated with potential infection, CSF evaluation is mandatory. In the acute setting of fever, meningismus, and encephalopathy, antimicrobial therapy should not be delayed while obtaining neuroimaging and lumbar puncture. Blood work, including blood cultures, should be obtained immediately. Regarding the collection of CSF, tube #1, the first tube of CSF collected, should not be the tube sent for Gram stain and culture and sensitivity because of possible skin or other procedural contamination.

There should be 0 polymorphonuclear leukocytes in the CSF and 5 or fewer lymphocytes. If the lumbar puncture is traumatic, the number can be adjusted by allowing 1 additional white blood cell (WBC) for each 700 red cells. In a traumatic tap with 7000 RBCs, the upper limit of normal CSF WBCs would be 5 + 7000/700, namely 12 WBCs. In differentiating bacterial from viral infection, the CSF glucose in relation to the serum glucose can be helpful. When the CSF glucose is reduced by 70% or more compared with the serum glucose, a bacterial infection is likely. For example, a CSF glucose of 15 mg/dL paired with a serum glucose of 100 mg/dL (85% reduction) strongly suggests a bacterial process.

Box 3 lists the CSF studies that I order routinely as well as those in situations that suggest acute meningitis presenting with headache or in immunocompromised patients. The combination of a normal MRI, a normal CSF opening pressure, and 0 cells in the CSF eliminates most of the serious causes of secondary headaches.

It does not eliminate the need for a targeted history, physical, and funduscopic examination.

In subarachnoid hemorrhage that is frequently preceded by sentinel bleeding, the CT, MRI, and CSF can be negative after 2 weeks. In the setting of a patient who had an extremely explosive, worst-ever headache several weeks ago that has yet to be evaluated and for which aneurysmal rupture is a concern, I recommend proceeding directly to the combination of MRI/MRA or CT/CTA depending on the advice of your local neuroradiologist.

Learn to do your own lumbar punctures, measure CSF pressure yourself, and start reviewing the neuroimaging studies (MRI and CT) of your patients. In time, this hands-on experience will build your confidence in identifying the causes of secondary headache, impart insight in differentiating high-quality from substandard work, and increase your professional interest in this critical but grossly underserved clinical problem. The evaluation of headaches can be interesting.

SUMMARY

Blood tests have a minor role in headache management and that role is limited to a few secondary headache conditions. In headache, as with any symptom, laboratory tests should be chosen based on solid clues derived from the targeted history and physical examination. A shotgun approach to blood tests that includes rare diseases or those with low local prevalence frequently yields false-positive results, which exposes the patient to the expense, anxiety, and risk inherent in misdiagnosis. Keep it simple and do not forget about spinal fluid (**Box 3**).

Factors That Cause Concern

Bernard M. Abrams, MD

KEYWORDS

- Red flags • Subarachnoid hemorrhage • Aneurysm • Space occupying lesion
- Meningitis • Cervical vessel dissection • Thunderclap headache

KEY POINTS

- Most headaches are benign, but vigilance for potential life-threatening conditions is mandatory.
- Knowledge of primary and secondary headaches is the starting point for differential diagnosis.
- Red flags include so-called first worst, increasing headaches, change in headaches, exertional headaches, and nocturnal headaches.
- Special conditions that merit concern are advanced age, prior history of serious medical conditions or cancer, diabetes mellitus, pregnancy, substance abuse, and psychiatric conditions.
- The history is the most important diagnostic tool.

Headaches are a common affliction and most have a benign import. However, physicians and patients alike often have significant concerns about them. The fear of having a brain tumor or aneurysm is often voiced by patients in clinical practice, especially if a relative or friend has had one of these conditions. How headaches that are benign be distinguished from those with life-threatening or disabling potential? The International Classification of Headache Disorders (ICHD-II), first published in 1988[1] and updated in the year 2004,[2,3] offers a new understanding of headache disorders. It is the key to the diagnosis and treatment of headaches. It divides headaches into primary and secondary, with 4 primary headache categories and 8 secondary headache categories. A primary headache disorder is not caused by another condition, whereas a secondary headache disorder is caused by another identifiable condition such as a brain tumor. For a headache to cause concern, it should fit into the secondary headache category. The current author classifies headaches as[4]:

- Acute, life threatening
- Chronic, life threatening
- Chronic, benign, non–life threatening

Dr Abrams has no disclosures.
Department of Neurology, University of Missouri School of Medicine-Kansas City, 2411 Holmes Street, Kansas City, Missouri MO 64106, USA
E-mail address: babrams@kc.rr.com

Med Clin N Am 97 (2013) 225–242
http://dx.doi.org/10.1016/j.mcna.2012.11.002
0025-7125/13/$ – see front matter © 2013 Elsevier Inc. All rights reserved.

Other potential subcategories are:

- Acute, benign
- Subacute, benign
- Subacute life threatening.

It is hoped that this approach will lend some additional clarity to the situation.

For many years, neurologists and internists have been called on to diagnose and treat individuals with headaches and, during that time, various sets of red flags or factors that cause concern have evolved. Few data exist on the prevalence of life-threatening or disabling conditions or even the prevalence of those headache conditions that have caused death or disability. A joint study from Tufts Medical Center in Boston, Massachusetts, and Beaumont Hospital in Ireland[5] recently characterized red flags retrospectively in 55 autopsied cases of sudden death associated with acute headache (**Table 1**). The most commonly associated red flag symptoms included age more than 50 years, loss of consciousness and collapse, and worst/thunderclap character of headache. Cause of death at autopsy comprised vascular events (60.4%), primary brain tumors/cysts (16.7%), and meningitis (6.25%). Aneurysms accounted for most of the vascular cases (22.9%), with loss of consciousness, occipital headache, neck pain, and a focal neurologic deficit seen more commonly in this subset of cases. In this limited series,[5] a tabulation of the red flags is instructive.

Various schemes and mnemonics have been proposed to facilitate separation into benign and life-threatening headaches. One such classification is the SNOOP mnemonic[6,7]:

S: systemic symptoms (fever, weight loss), secondary risks (human immunodeficiency virus [HIV], cancer)
N: neurologic symptoms/signs (altered consciousness, focal deficits)
O: onset: sudden or split second (suggests subarachnoid hemorrhage)
O: older: new or progressive in a patient more than 50 years old (suggests temporal arteritis)

Table 1
Red flags associated with sudden death in acute headache

Red Flag Feature	N (Total = 55)	Percentage
Headache >50 y	30	54.54
Seizure/collapse/LOC	29	52.72
Thunderclap	28	51
Worst headache	25	45.5
Drowsy/confused/agitated	18	32.7
Progressive visual/neurologic symptoms	18	32.7
Nausea/vomiting	17	30.9
Paralysis/weakness/Babinski sign	12	21.8
Sensory loss	7	12.7
Meningeal irritation	6	10.9
Associated systemic illness[a]	6	10.9
Pupil asymmetry	5	9.09
Ataxia/incoordination	I	1.08

Abbreviation: LOC, loss of consciousness.
[a] Pyrexia, night sweats, respiratory distress, pneumonia.

P: prior history: first, newly progressive, or different from usual headache; positional (suggests abnormal spinal fluid pressure); papilledema (think mass lesion, increased intracranial pressure [ICP])

A patient-oriented mnemonic is HPAIN. Although its primary purpose is to alert patients to possible secondary causes of headaches and increase awareness, it is informative even for physicians.[8]

H stands for the host (the patient). Is the patient more than 50 years old? Does the patient have cancer, HIV, heart disease, or diabetes? Is the patient at risk for other illness? Is the patient on immunosuppressant drug therapy? Does the patient smoke? If the patient has an underlying medical process and then suddenly has a headache that the patient has never experienced before, it could suggest a dangerous complication caused by medication or the underlying disease process.

P stands for pattern. Is this the same old headache or a change from what the patient is used to? Are the headaches escalating rapidly or has one developed that just will not quit? Has there been abrupt onset? Is this a new and unusual headache, a thunderclap felt in the head followed by the worst pain that the patient has ever experienced? A headache that comes on in a matter of seconds and may be caused by a ruptured brain aneurysm.

A stands for the associated signs or symptoms. Is this more than just a headache or does it come with anything else such as fever, stiff neck, chills, or weight loss? The patient may have viral or bacterial meningitis, and infection of the meninges that cover the brain.

I is for anything unusual that increases the pain. Any unusual features are of interest here: did it occur for the first time after recent intercourse? Does sleep bring it on or make it worse? Did it begin after a head injury? Is this pain provoked by lifting, coughing, standing, or yelling?

N is for any neurologic signs or symptoms. Is there any weakness, numbness, blindness, or difficulty with speech, or has there been a seizure? The patient may have suffered a stroke or have a tumor or abscess.

RED FLAGS FOR SECONDARY HEADACHES
Sudden Onset of a Headache: the First, Worst Headache, Thunderclap Headache, Sentinel Headache (Acute, Life Threatening)

Here the concern is that the patient reports that a severe headache is of sudden onset, especially if it is the first occurrence of that type of headache. There is the possibility of a subarachnoid hemorrhage, bleeding from an arteriovenous malformation or a mass lesion, especially in the posterior fossa (**Fig. 1**). Other causes include cervical artery dissection, venous sinus thrombosis, and pituitary apoplexy.

Investigation in these circumstances is mandatory and neuroimaging, usually computed tomography (CT), is indicated. A lumbar puncture following imaging may be indicated to rule out an infectious process or bleeding not detected by the primary imaging technique. Any chronic primary headache such as migraine must have an initial event, and this often produces confusion in the emergency room.

The age, physical condition of the patient, past medical history, and family history play a strong role in deciding what to do, although imaging is often done. A child or young adult with a strong family history of migraine should cause less concern that a previously headache-free individual who is 50 years old.

This category includes thunderclap headache. A sudden severe headache may have serious import and may be a primary thunderclap headache. Vascular causes include subarachnoid hemorrhage, aneurysmal thrombosis or expansion, cervical

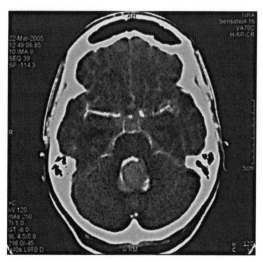

Fig. 1. Contrast cranial CT scan. There is hyperdense blood within the basal cisterns and subarachnoid spaces, revealing severe subarachnoid hemorrhage. (*From* Horisberger T, Lorenzana D, Noethiger CB, et al. Isolated noncompaction of the ventricular myocardium in a patient presenting with subarachnoid hemorrhage. Int J Cardiol 2007;116(3):e98–100; with permission.)

arterial dissection, reversible cerebral vasoconstriction syndrome, cerebral venous thrombosis, hypertensive crisis, pituitary apoplexy, or retroclival hematoma. Nonvascular causes include spontaneous intracranial hypotension or hypovolemia, meningitis, sphenoid sinusitis, and colloid cyst of the third ventricle, but may also include benign conditions such as primary cough, sexual and exertional headache, or primary thunderclap headache (**Fig. 2**).[7] As with almost all headaches, imaging should be performed before lumbar puncture but lumbar puncture is necessary to check for evidence of bleeding and to check cerebrospinal fluid (CSF) pressure. Magnetic resonance (MR) angiography or CT angiography can exclude dissection, reversible cerebral vasoconstriction syndrome (RCVS), or unruptured aneurysm. MR venography or CT venography can identify cerebral venous thrombosis. MR imaging with gadolinium and general medical evaluation can reveal most other causes of thunderclap headache.[8] A negative work-up indicates a probable diagnosis of primary thunderclap headache. The so-called sentinel headache remains one of the most discussed premonitory symptoms of subarachnoid hemorrhage and a potent source of malpractice suits after emergency room encounters. The value of a lumbar puncture, even after a normal CT scan, is almost incontrovertible at this point,[9] although its value has been questioned by some.[10]

Exceptions to the First, Worst Rule

In the classification discussed earlier,[4] the terms acute and life threatening are used. Not all patients with headache who are seen in the emergency room have life-threatening conditions. Acute, non–life-threatening conditions are frequently met, even in the setting of first, worst, in which the headache is the first in a series of benign chronic headaches. Migraine headaches can be extremely severe and are categorized by more than 80% of sufferers as severe to extremely severe. Factors that give reassurance are age less than 25 years; strong family history of migraine in a first-degree relative; a classic aura of visual scotoma, especially scintillating with the onset of

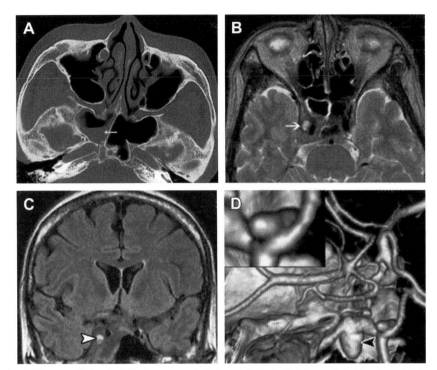

Fig. 2. Neuroradiological findings on admission. (*A*) Brain CT showed right sphenoid sinusitis (*thin arrow*) and no bony deficit. (*B*) T2-weighted magnetic resonance imaging (MRI) revealed a high-intensity small round lesion (*thick arrow*) and enlargement of the right cavernous sinus. (*C*) There was no enhancement in the right cavernous sinus in the coronal section of T1-weighted MRI with gadolinium diethylenetriaminepentaacetic acid (Gd-DTPA) (*white arrowhead*), although the left side was enhanced. (*D*) Three-dimensional computed tomographic angiography revealed 2 aneurysms; 1 was located in the cavernous portion of the internal carotid artery (*black arrowhead*) and the other in the internal carotid-posterior communicating (IC-PC) portion (inset). (*From* Sugie M, Ihihara K, Nakano I, et al. Infectious aneurysm of the intracavernous carotid artery occurring concomitantly with sphenoid sinusitis; an autopsy case report. J Neurol Sci 2009;278(1–2):115–8.)

headache 20 minutes to 1 hour later; and a strong history of childhood antecedents of migraine with carsickness, motion sickness, cyclic vomiting, or unexplained vertigo. A history of precipitating events including alcohol ingestion, ingestion of substances containing tyramine, prolonged sleeplessness, or conditions leading to hypoglycemia should be considered.

Although routine imaging in children has been decried by some, prudence dictates caution. Although migraines are the most common cause of headaches in children, it is important to be aware of other, secondary causes of headaches. Secondary headaches have an underlying cause that may be systemic (medical) or a problem inherent in the central nervous system. Common intracranial causes for headache in children include structural causes (eg, tumor, hydrocephalus, Chiari malformation), infection (encephalitis or meningitis), inflammatory causes (acute disseminated encephalomyelitis, multiple sclerosis, vasculitis), and epilepsy (**Fig. 3**). In some situations, early identification and appropriate treatment of these underlying conditions can result in complete headache resolution. Seizures may have headaches as a prominent feature.[11–13]

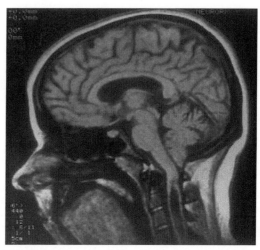

Fig. 3. Midsagittal T1-weighted image. Note the typical features of the Chiari I malformation: tonsillar ectopia below C1 level, absence of cisterna magna, and a syringomyelia (low-signal area in the central region of the spinal cord). (*From* Haouzi P, Marchal J, Allioui EM, et al. Corticospinal pathway and exercise hyperpnea: lessons from a patient with Arnold Chiari malformation. Respir Physiol 2000;123(1–2):13–22; with permission.)

A worsening headache pattern (subacute or chronic, benign, or life threatening) causes concern for a mass lesion, subdural hematoma (especially after trauma), or medication overuse and/or rebound. The past headache history is key. If there is a long-standing headache disorder that has worsened, this suggests:

1. The development of a superimposed headache disorder (either primary or secondary), or
2. A primary preexisting headache disorder becoming chronic

Risk factors for primary headaches such as migraine or tension-type headaches becoming chronic include high frequency of headaches, overuse of acute medications, obesity, stressful life events, alcohol overuse, hypothyroidism, viral infections, head trauma, snoring, and sleep disturbances. The most common reason for an episodic headache to become chronic is medication overuse. Another article written by Dr. Bernard M. Abrams in this issue covers this important subject in detail.

The setting of the headache and the physical state and past medical history of the patient are often a clue to the possible nature of this type of headache. Neuroimaging, a careful history of medication intake, and possibly a drug screen are indicated. In this instance, MR imaging (MRI) is usually superior to CT scanning.

Several factors heighten concern: age of onset more than 50 years, worsening pattern of frequency of intensity in a new-onset headache, and prior history of a condition that may affect the brain (discussed later) including cancer, immunosuppression such as for acquired immune deficiency syndrome (AIDS)/HIV, or conditions predisposing to trauma, and occult trauma, especially alcoholism, substance abuse, and dementia.

Headache associated with systemic illness (acute benign, acute life threatening, subacute life threatening) is a further cause for concern. Many systemic disorders are associated with a prominent complaint of acute headache, including:

1. Intracranial and extracranial infections (meningitis, encephalitis, Lyme disease, HIV, sinusitis)

2. Hypoxia and hypercapnia (high-altitude illness, diving, sleep apnea)
3. Dialysis-uncontrolled arterial hypertension, hypotension, hypothyroidism, fasting
4. Collagen-vascular disorders, systemic arteritis
5. Carbon monoxide poisoning

However, especially in subacute or chronic headaches, the condition may be occult and a high index of suspicion is required. Thinking outside the headache realm and a complete history, review of systems, and thorough physical examination are requisite. The manifestations of systemic diseases are protean and include (but are by no means limited to) fever, rash, joint pain or swelling, weight loss or gain, and change in bowel or bladder habits. Diagnostic considerations include cancer,[14] infections,[15] and opportunistic infection in an immunocompromised host. Immunocompromised hosts include patients with cancer patients on chemotherapy, and patients with HIV/AIDS complex or diabetes. Investigations required may include neuroimaging, collagen-vascular evaluation, lumbar puncture, immune status work-up, or infectious disease work-up. Any systemic manifestation in conjunction with a headache should occasion concern.

Secondary Headache Entities Associated with Laboratory Abnormalities

Blood and urine tests are helpful in certain systemic disorders causing headaches.[16] Two rare disorders are Cerebral autosomal dominant arteriopathy with subcortical infarcts and leukoencephalopathy (CADASIL) and mitochondrial encephalomyopathy, lactic acidosis, and strokelike episodes (MELAS) (**Fig. 4**).

CADASIL is a single-gene disorder that affects small vessels in the brain. The diagnosis is suggested by attacks of migraine with aura occurring in association with

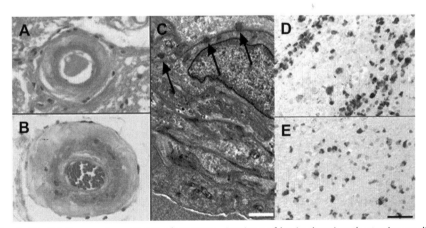

Fig. 4. (*A, B*) Microscopic evidence of CADASIL. Sections of brain showing the tunica media of cerebral parenchymal (*A*) and leptomeningeal (*B*) arterioles that are replaced by poorly defined granular eosinophilic material. There is also adventitial fibrosis. (*C*) Electron microscopy of a dermal arteriole reveals collections of granular osmiophilic material (*arrows*) adjacent to vascular smooth muscle cells. The appearances are typical of CADASIL. (*D, E*) Microscopic evidence of multiple system atrophy. Sections of putamen (*D*) and internal capsule (*E*) that have been labeled for α-synuclein contain numerous glial cytoplasmic inclusions as well as occasional immunopositive neuronal inclusions. Bar = 100 μm in A, B, D, and E; 1 μm in C. (*From* Rice CM, McGuone D, Kurian KM, et al. Autopsy-confirmed, co-existent CADASIL and multiple system atrophy. Parkinsonism Relat Disord 2011;17(5):390–2; with permission.)

characteristic multiple confluent white matter lesions shown on brain MRI. Blood can be sent for genetic testing to identify NOTCH 3 mutations on chromosome 19. ICHD-II requires diagnostic confirmation of CADASIL with either skin biopsy or genetic testing.

MELAS should be suspected in patients who have attacks of migraine in conjunction with seizures or strokelike episodes. It is a mitochondrial disorder with maternal inheritance. Blood tests may show increased levels of lactate and pyruvate in the serum, but these abnormalities do not confirm the diagnosis. Blood can be sent for genetic testing for MELAS point mutations. ICHD-II requires demonstration of a MELAS point mutation, but can be accomplished without a blood test. Genetic testing can also be performed on skeletal muscle samples, hair follicles, urine sediment, or mucosal biopsy specimens. Mucosal biopsy specimens may be more reliable than leukocyte testing.

Headache Attributed to Intracranial Hypertension Secondary to Metabolic, Toxic, or Hormonal Causes

Blood tests can be used to assess levels of vitamin A or endocrine disorders; urine tests can detect use of anabolic steroids.[17]

Headache Attributed to Other Noninfectious Inflammatory Diseases

Blood tests for autoantibodies (antibody to nuclear antigens, anti-SM, anti–double-stranded DNA) can help establish a diagnosis of systemic lupus erythematosus. Anemia, thrombocytopenia, or leukopenia may also be diagnostic clues. Urine testing may show proteinuria consistent with renal involvement in lupus. ICHD-II criteria require evidence of an inflammatory disease known to be associated with headache; for most such disorders, blood tests are useful.

Headache Attributed to Hypothalamic or Pituitary Hypersecretion or Hyposecretion

Blood tests may show abnormalities of prolactin, growth hormone, or adrenocorticotropic hormone. ICHD-II criteria for this diagnosis can also be met by demonstration of abnormalities of temperature regulation, emotions, or thirst in association with a tumor.

Headache Attributed to Substances or Their Withdrawal

Blood and urine tests may be needed to document the presence of the suspected drug or toxin. These substances include mercury, copper, lead, alcohol, marijuana, and cocaine. ICHD-II criteria do not specify that testing is necessary for diagnosis, but specify that use of the offending substance must be established.

Headaches Attributed to Bacterial, Viral, or Other Systemic Infection

Blood or urine tests may help identify the cause of the infection or accompanying inflammation.[15] ICHD-II criteria requires testing to identify the bacterial organism and show evidence of viral or other infection, but do not specify the tests that must be used.

Headache Attributed to HIV Infection

Rapid screening tests for HIV can be performed on blood or oral fluid samples; positive tests must be confirmed with a venous blood sample evaluated for antibodies to the retrovirus using immunoassay procedures. Tests may be negative in early infection during a window period of 2 to 8 weeks. About half of infected patients experience headache during acute seroconversion, with a mean duration of 26 days.

Blood testing is required to meet ICHD-II criteria for a diagnosis of headache attributed to HIV infection. ICHD-II criteria distinguish this headache from that caused by other viral infections and comment that "dull bilateral headache may be a part of the symptomatology of HIV infection." Diagnosis of this headache requires blood testing for confirmation of HIV infection.

Headache Attributed to Disorders of Homeostasis

Blood or urine tests are useful to diagnose many of these headache disorders.[17] A 24-hour urine sample for creatinine, total catecholamines, vanillylmandelic acid, and metaneprines has a good balance of sensitivity and specificity; plasma testing for metanephrine levels is the most sensitive test. Thyroid-stimulating hormone and thyroxine levels can establish a diagnosis of hypothyroidism. Urine testing for proteinuria is needed when preeclampsia is suspected.

ICHD-II criteria require demonstration of proteinuria for diagnosis of preeclampsia or eclampsia. A diagnosis of headache attributed to hypothyroidism also requires blood testing. In contrast, although characteristic findings on blood tests can establish a diagnosis of pheochromocytoma, this can also be based on surgical or imaging findings in combination with other features such as hypertension.[16]

Headache associated with focal neurologic signs (acute, subacute, or chronic, life threatening) should lead to consideration of a mass lesion, vascular lesion, arteriovenous malformation, or collagen-vascular disorder. The differential diagnosis of headache plus focal findings is broad and the work-up should be guided by the patient's profile of other risk factors. A first differential characteristic is whether the neurologic signs or symptoms are transient or persistent. Transient signs are less significant if there is an obvious visual or sensory aura for migraine, usually followed within 20 minutes to an hour with a headache. Familiarity in this case gives a sense of security that there is a primary headache disorder. If an aura or focal neurologic signs persist following the cessation of the headache, neuroimaging and other investigations are indicated.

Focal neurologic signs other than migraine aura demand investigation, although it is common to be confused about long-standing and irrelevant findings such as infantile hemiparesis, absent reflexes, diminished sensation, or motor weakness caused by lower motor neuron disease such as radiculopathies and carpal tunnel syndrome.

Focal neurologic signs may indicate a mass lesion including primary brain tumors, metastatic brain tumors, abscesses, and vascular lesions such as arteriovenous malformation or collagen-vascular disorder. Neuroimaging is a first step with collagen-vascular evaluation and other laboratory data become relevant according to circumstances.[16] Cervical artery dissection requires dedicated imaging of the cervical arteries, whereas cerebral venous sinus thrombosis requires dedicated imaging of the cerebral venous system. Idiopathic intracranial hypertension requires the measurement of cerebral spinal fluid pressure. Infections, such as cryptococcal meningitis or Lyme meningitis, require spinal fluid analysis.

Abnormal optic fundi findings such as papilledema lead to consideration of a mass lesion,[18] pseudotumor cerebri (benign intracranial hypertension), hypertensive crisis, encephalitis, or meningitis. A work-up is indicated including neuroimaging and lumbar puncture (almost always done after neuroimaging), as well as appropriate laboratory tests.

Headache associated with personality or cognitive changes raises questions of chronic brain lesions such as tumor (especially frontal), subdural hematoma, chronic meningitis, or other chronic general medical problem and requires neuroimaging and further tests dictated by the patient's general medical condition.

Headache Triggered by Cough, Exertion, or Orgasm

These are triggered headaches, severe headaches unequivocally triggered by cough, heavy exercise, or orgasm. Postcoital headaches, mild headaches following exercise, and mild headaches followed by cough do not seem to be associated with secondary headaches at a higher risk than headaches not associated with red flags.[7] This article presents the differentiation between sexual headaches as described by Matthew and Garza.[19]

Primary preorgasmic headache, as occurring during sexual activity and increasing with sexual excitement and state, is less worrisome for secondary causes compared with orgasmic headache.

Orgasmic headaches occur at orgasm, are typically thunderclap headaches, and may have secondary causes such as subarachnoid hemorrhage, arterial dissection, or CSF leak. On the first occasion, work-up is mandatory. Donnet and colleagues[20] conducted a clinical and radiological study of cough headache, primary exertional headache, and headache associated with sexual activity. Results were analyzed for 41 patients. In 19 patients, headaches were associated with sexual activity (8 preorgasmic and 12 orgasmic). Venous stenosis was noted in 12/19 but the results remain controversial.

Exertional headaches may be primary, as in migraine or primary exertional headache, or secondary, as in subarachnoid headache, intracranial neoplasm, third ventricle colloid cyst, arterial dissection, pheochromocytoma, or cardiac ischemia.[19]

Headache triggered by straining, coughing, or sneezing suggests posterior fossa disease including hindbrain malformation, occipitocervical junction disorder (including Arnold-Chiari malformation),[7] or increased ICP. There may be a CSF leak or an intracranial aneurysm. About 50% have primary cough headache.[19] MRI, MR angiography (MRA), and MR venography (MRV) are mandatory. These headaches are usually brief and about 50% have structural causes.[6] Six of 7 patients with primary cough headaches[20] had venous stenosis, 3 in the transverse sinuses and 3 in the jugular veins. Again, these results are preliminary and controversial, dictating caution in interpreting newer radiological studies until further data are received.

Headache During Pregnancy or Postpartum

Most headaches that occur during pregnancy or postpartum are primary migraine or tension-type headaches, although generally migraine headaches are significantly less frequent during pregnancy.[21] In a pregnant or postpartum woman with a history of migraine or tension-type headache, without atypical features and with a normal examination, investigation is usually not necessary.[7] However, some women report new onset of severe headaches with migraine features, or a worsening pattern of a previously diagnosed primary headache. In these cases, cortical vein or cranial sinus thrombosis, carotid dissection, and pituitary apoplexy enter into the differential diagnosis. These disorders are more common in the third trimester or in the early postpartum period. Stroke is thought to be more common in late pregnancy and the early postpartum period. Neuroimaging, including MRI and MRA, is necessary to exclude such vascular disorders. The differential diagnosis also includes preeclampsia, a multisystem disorder with various forms. In addition to hypertension and proteinuria, tissue edema, thrombocytopenia, and abnormalities in liver function can occur. Preeclampsia seems to involve a strong maternal inflammatory response with broad systemic activity. Subsidiary investigation includes blood and urine testing.[7,16]

Positional Headaches

Orthostatic and reverse-orthostatic headaches may indicate disorders of the CSF pathways or dynamics.[19] Although orthostatic headaches are typically caused by low pressure/volume, and reverse-orthostatic headaches can be caused by increased pressure/volume, the opposite may also be true. Increased pressure/volume usually does not present with positional headaches, but rather with visual changes, pulsatile tinnitus, and papilledema, with variable headache quality. The diagnosis of a low pressure/volume state is suggested not only by orthostatic headache but also by onset later in the day. Migraine features are common, and, if significant hindbrain descent occurs, cerebellar and brainstem signs and symptoms may be present. MRI with gadolinium may show brain sag, pituitary engorgement, and pachymeningeal enhancement, and MRV may show the venous distention sign of a convex appearance to the transverse sinuses on sagittal view. Some orthostatic headaches are caused by slow, undetectable leaks or result from increased compliance of the lower lumbar CSF space without leak. Other orthostatic headaches are not caused by CSF pressure dysregulation, but by autonomic dysfunction in disorders such as orthostatic hypotension.[22]

Headache in the Elderly

Headache in this age group should always be investigated for secondary causes, although primary headaches do occur. Giant cell arteritis is an underdiagnosed and preventable cause of visual loss in the elderly. When giant cell arteritis is suspected (headache, constitutional signs and symptoms, jaw claudication, temporal artery tenderness), erythrocyte sedimentation rate (ESR) and C-reactive peptide (CRP) levels should be obtained. The absence of abnormalities of ESR or CRP abnormalities does not preclude the diagnosis and a biopsy of the temporal artery should be obtained to seek characteristic granulomatous inflammatory lesions.

Common diagnostic considerations are cervicogenic headache from severe degenerative disease, metastatic cancer, and subdural hemorrhage; these are usually suggested by typical history and examination findings. A common primary headache disorder in the elderly is hypnic headache, which is discussed later.

Headaches Associated with Sleep or Awakening from Sleep

Secondary headaches include intracranial space–occupying lesions, increased ICP, idiopathic intracranial hypertension (pseudotumor cerebri), medication-overuse headache, obstructive sleep apnea, and cervicogenic headaches. Primary headaches include hypnic headaches, cluster headaches and migraines.

Hypnic headache is a primary headache characterized by short-lived headaches that occur exclusively during sleep. ICHD-II (Headache Classification Subcommittee of the International Headache Society 2004) officially defines hypnic headache. The criteria require a dull headache without autonomic symptoms and no more than 1 of the following symptoms: nausea, photophobia, or phonophobia. At least 2 of the following characteristics are also required: occurrence greater than or equal to 15 times a month, duration greater than 15 minutes after awakening, and first occurrence after the age of 50 years.[2] Cluster headache usually occurs during the first rapid eye movement sleep cycle about 90 minutes after retiring and then recurring about every 45 minutes. Migraine is irregularly associated with sleep and many sufferers awaken with a migraine headache. Because migraine and cluster are so well defined as primary headache types they are not discussed further here.

APPLICATION OF A HISTORY-TAKING SCHEME TO IDENTIFY FACTORS THAT ARE CONCERNING

The author has advanced a series of questions in the general context of headache diagnosis.[4] An article in this issue covers the general headache history but certain questions have particular relevance to factors that cause concern. The full list is given here and some of them are discussed in detail later.

1. Where am I?
2. What is the matter?
3. Has this ever happened before?
4. If this has happened before, is it progressive?
5. If this has happened before, for how long, and has it changed?
6. If it is the same, what is the pattern of occurrence?
7. What is the character and location?
8. What is the onset-to-peak time?
9. What is the usual time of day when it occurs and the total duration?
10. Are there any associated and/or residual neurologic phenomena or sequelae?
11. Is there an aura?
12. What makes the headache worse?
13. What makes the headache better?
14. Is there a family history?
15. Were there headaches in childhood?
16. Was there motion sickness, cyclical vomiting, dizziness, or unexplained fever in childhood?
17. Were there any prior diagnostic tests?
18. What were the results of prior medication?
19. Are there any other medical illnesses?
20. Are there any psychiatric illnesses or history of alcohol or substance abuse, and what is the quality of the individual's life?

The order selected for these questions is important, because it accomplishes in the briefest period of time and in the most economical manner the goals of separating headaches; first, into those that may present an acute, life-threatening situation; and, second, into those that are chronic or benign.

Question 1: Where am I?

Although this may seem like a frivolous question designed to test the examiner's sense of orientation, it is the beginning of a separation of headaches into 1 or 2 types. A clinician in the emergency room sees a patient in 2 types of situations: (1) an acute, life-threatening situation; or (2) the first chronic benign headache that is severe. Life-threatening headaches present as either headaches of great severity associated with meningeal signs, which immediately suggests the need for contrast studies, usually an immediate CT scan followed by a lumbar puncture; or focal hemispheric-type syndromes giving unilateral signs, symptoms, and, perhaps, signs of increased ICP.

Confusion arises with the first chronic benign headache, such as a migraine headache in a 15-year-old girl. Therefore the clinician may have to go through the differential diagnosis and also do everything required of an acute life-threatening headache to rule out any life-threatening problem. The first headache of a chronic, benign sequence that is a sufficiently severe migraine, cluster, or muscle-contraction headache; trigeminal neuralgia; sinusitis; and many other types of headaches may lead the first-time sufferer to the emergency room, whereas, with repeated familiarity, the patient seeks the appropriate treatment.

If the physician is in the hospital as a consultant, then it may be an acute or chronic life-threatening situation that has gone beyond the emergency-room stage. In the emergency room, all immediately demonstrable life-threatening headaches will presumably have been resolved so that the CT scan shows a subarachnoid hemorrhage, tumor, or cerebral edema, and the lumbar puncture has ruled in or out any type of meningeal syndrome, most likely infection or subarachnoid hemorrhage.

Question 2 is nonspecific but may convey information about the condition, including thunderclap headaches.

Question 3: Has this Ever Happened Before?

The initial 3-question sequence is crucial to separating acute and chronic and benign or primary headaches from secondary and potentially life-threatening ones. Headaches that have recurred over a significant period of time with a familiar pattern are more likely primary entities such as migraine or tension-type headaches in spite of their severity. Even a first-time headache may be the start of a primary benign disorder but this is unknowable at that point.

Question 4: If this has Happened Before, is it Progressive?

This speaks to the differentiation between subacute or chronic (depending on length and continuous or intermittent nature). An inexorable increase in headache frequency and intensity, especially in conjunction with other warning signs, such as new-onset headache recently in the elderly, immunocompromised, or an individual with a history of cancer known to metastasize to the brain, is an obvious source of concern, whereas a lifelong migraine sufferer with an increased frequency and intensity may have chronification through several factors, the most common of which is medication-overuse headache.

Question 5: If this has Happened Before, for How Long, and has it Changed?

This is a corollary to question 4, giving a temporal and qualitative quality to the previous question, and it speaks to whether the problem is intermittent (less likely to be life threatening) or continuous, and how its frequency, intensity, location, and character have changed.

Questions 6 and 7: If it is the Same, What is the Pattern of Occurrence? What is the Character and Location?

These questions are most appropriate for determining the description of chronic benign headaches which, reassuringly, have stayed the same over time.

Question 8: What is the Onset-to-peak Time?

This question has the greatest significance in an acute headache, especially a first-time occurrence, which, coupled with the intensity, may indicate a thunderclap headache. Once established that the headache is not life threatening, it gives some differential information among primary headache types because migraine usually peaks faster than tension-type headaches, 20 minutes to 2 hours versus 4 to 6 hours, and longer than cluster headaches, which are usually around 15 minutes or less.

Question 9: What is the Usual Time of Day When it Occurs and the Total Duration?

Although increased ICP is the most alarming possible cause of nocturnal and/or awakening headaches, the sensitivity and specificity of this symptom for the diagnosis of intracranial hypertension has not been systematically evaluated. ICHD-II lists only 2 categories in which headache that is worst in the morning is included among the diagnostic criteria, namely headache attributed directly to neoplasm' and headache attributed to intracranial hypertension secondary to hydrocephalus.[23] However, morning headaches may occur with other causes of increased ICP; for example, the headache of idiopathic intracranial hypertension may awaken the patient at night.[24] Nocturnal and/or awakening headache is not a pathognomonic symptom for increased ICP. Many other headache disorders enter the differential diagnosis, some common such as migraine, as well as other neurologic and medical conditions. Using this or another history-taking method is key to identifying them **(Box 1)**.[24,25]

Box 1
Differential diagnosis of nocturnal and/or awakening headaches

Primary headache disorders (benign, usually chronic)

    Migraine

    Trigeminal autonomic cephalalgias (includes cluster)

    Cluster headache

    Paroxysmal hemicrania

    Short-lasting unilateral neuralgiform headaches with conjunctival injection and tearing

    Hemicrania continua

    Hypnic headache

    Primary headache associated with sexual activity

Secondary headache disorders (life threatening, acute, subacute, or chronic)

    Increased ICP

    Neoplasm

    Intracranial hypertension secondary to hydrocephalus

    Secondary headache disorders

    Medication-overuse headache

    Hangover headache

    Giant cell (temporal) arteritis

    Sphenoid sinusitis

    Carbon monoxide–induced headache

    Subarachnoid hemorrhage

    Headache attributed to epileptic seizure

    Sleep apnea hypopnea headache

    Depression

    Exploding head syndrome[a]

[a] This may be regarded as a physiologic phenomenon in the transition from wakefulness to sleep, akin to nocturnal myoclonus.[25,26]

Adapted from Larner AJ. Not all morning headaches are due to brain tumor. Pract Neurol 2009;9:80–4.

Question 10: Are There any Associated and/or Residual Neurologic Phenomena or Sequelae?

The most usual neurologic phenomenon associated with a headache is the scintillating scotoma or sensory abnormality of migraine, which usually subsides as the headache evolves or shortly thereafter. Any persistence of neurologic symptoms or signs beyond that warrants a work-up. Neurologic symptoms or signs between headaches signify the possibility of a life-threatening condition.

Question 11: Is There an Aura?

This question is specific for migraine with aura. Repeatable aura, especially for more than a few attacks, should be reassuring.[2]

Questions 12 and 13: What Makes the Headache Worse? What Makes the Headache Better?

This question may yield valuable information about the possibility of a life-threatening condition if factors such as aggravation by Valsalva maneuvers or head position are present, but benign conditions such as migraine of tension-type headache are often aggravated by hypoglycemia, lack of sleep and vasoactive foods, stress, and other factors. Life-threatening headaches may be ameliorated, at least early in their course, by seemingly innocuous remedies such as aspirin, acetaminophen, and nonsteroidal antiinflammatory drugs, giving the impression that they are benign. Benign headaches are often relieved by measures such as ice packs, a dark room, and sleep. All headaches may be helped by opioids and other controlled substances.

Questions 14, 15, and 16: Is There a Family History? Were There Headaches in Childhood? Was There Motion Sickness, Cyclical Vomiting, Dizziness, or Unexplained Fever in Childhood?

This trio of questions relates largely to the diagnosis of migraines because these are all factors leading, if positive, toward that diagnosis. These questions carry little weight in differentiating benign from life-threatening headaches because their specificity for this common benign class of headaches is high but the sensitivity in the early questioning is low because a secondary headache type could coexist with migraines, which affect about12% of the total population. Hence, the questions are asked only after the probability of a secondary headache is low and the examiner needs to confirm which type of primary headache disorder is present.

Question 17: Were There any Prior Diagnostic Tests?

Although this question is self-explanatory, it deserves some discussion. If a determination is made of a primary benign headache disorder, the injunction against unnecessary testing of the patient holds, but it leaves the dilemma of what to do with the patient who presents more than once with atypical headaches or even repeated thunderclap headaches. Can subarachnoid hemorrhage be missed by not reimaging patients who present on numerous occasions? Cerebrovascular aneurysms are present in 2% of the population,[6] whereas national data reveal that 30,000 Americans suffer a subarachnoid hemorrhage each year.[7]

Aneurysmal subarachnoid hemorrhage is a devastating illness, with mortality approaching 50% and substantial morbidity.[27,28]

Noncontrast head CT diagnoses most cases of subarachnoid hemorrhage, particularly if performed soon after it occurs. The sensitivity of head CT for subarachnoid blood decreases with time because the hemoglobin within the CSF is metabolized and diluted. If performed within 6 hours, the sensitivity of head CT approaches

100%, although this diminishes to 90% to 95% by 24 hours and less than 75% within several days. To exclude the diagnosis of subarachnoid hemorrhage definitively, a spinal fluid analysis is required to find evidence of bleeding. This evidence may be in the form of red blood cells not attributable to trauma from the lumbar puncture, or xanthochromia, the yellowish tinge that CSF acquires from the metabolism of red blood cells. Xanthochromia may take hours to develop, so a lumbar puncture within several hours of the bleed may not show xanthochromia. As an alternative, rather than a lumbar puncture, a CT angiogram or MR angiogram may be used to evaluate for a causative aneurysm. Although these imaging modalities are not 100% sensitive for causative aneurysms, the combination of either of these tests with a normal non-contrast head CT is sufficiently sensitive. MR angiogram can locate an aneurysm and a lumbar puncture can identify blood in the CSF.[29] However, with these parameters, there is still a dilemma as to whether, by virtue of bad timing, a subarachnoid hemorrhage could have been missed (**Box 2**).

Question 18: What Were the Results of Prior Medication?

Medication-overuse headache may occur. Although largely used for assessing the efficacy of medications and adjusting medications in known conditions, this question affords an opportunity to find out about medication overuse. Near the end of questioning, a patient is more comfortable with the physician and likely to give a reliable answer. This time is also suitable to inquire about other medications (vasoactive

---

Box 2
Canadian subarachnoid decision rule

Each of these 3 rules was 100% sensitive for identifying subarachnoid hemorrhage in a population of patients with nontraumatic headache that peaked in intensity within 1 hour. These rules have yet to be validated in a distinct population.

Rule 1

    Older than 40 years

    Complaint of neck pain or stiffness

    Witnessed loss of consciousness

    Onset with exertion

Rule 2

    Arrival by ambulance

    Older than 45 years

    Vomiting at least once

    Diastolic blood pressure greater than 100 mm Hg

Rule 3

    Arrival by ambulance

    Systolic blood pressure greater than 160 mm Hg

    Complaint of neck pain or stiffness

    Aged 45 to 55 years

Modified from Perry JJ, Stiell IG, Sivilotti ML, et al. High risk clinical characteristics for subarachnoid hemorrhage in patients with acute headache: prospective cohort study. BMJ 2010;341:c5204; with permission.

substances, indocin, and others) that may cause headaches on their own. An inquiry about industrial and home exposures to potential headache-causing circumstances is also in order at this time.

Question 19: Are There any Other Medical Illnesses?

This is an important question for reasons that are obvious.

Question 20: Is There any History of Psychiatric Disorder, Substance Abuse, or Litigation?

The reason for reserving these questions for last is that by now patients should be convinced of the interest of the physician in their welfare. Introduction of these questions early in questioning may be viewed as pejorative. A substantial, but unknown, proportion of acute, subacute, and chronic headaches are related to depression and anxiety. A smaller number are related to personality disorders. A history of prior substance abuse raises a red flag, although recovery is known among substance abusers who may then be subject to both primary and secondary headache disorders.

THE PHYSICAL AND NEUROLOGIC EXAMINATION

Elsewhere in this issue there is an article on the targeted headache examination. Deviations from normal (with the exception of papilledema) may be related or unrelated and relevant or not. A careful history prepares the examiner for these variations.

SUMMARY

Headaches can be benign or life threatening but, with careful attention to the details described in this article, the correct diagnosis and treatment can be arrived at in many cases. Modern imaging techniques have taken the guesswork out of many conditions but a high index of suspicion and attention to red flags helps avoid potential adverse outcomes in headache encounters in a high proportion of cases.

REFERENCES

1. Headache Classification Committee of the International Headache Society. Classification and diagnostic criteria for headache disorders, cranial neuralgia, and facial pain. Cephalalgia 1988;8:1–96.
2. Headache Classification Committee of the International Headache Society. The international classification of headache disorders. Cephalalgia 2004;24(Suppl 1): 1–160.
3. Olesen J, Lipton RB. Headache classification update 2004. Curr Opin Neurol 2004;17:275–82.
4. Abrams BM. Tutorial 29: evaluation and treatment of common headache syndromes. Pain Digest 1997;7:92–103.
5. Lynch KM, Brett F. Headaches that kill: a retrospective study of incidence, clinical features in cases of sudden death. Cephalalgia 2012;32(13):972–8.
6. Dodick DW. Clinical clues and clinical rules: primary vs secondary headache. Adv Stud Med 2003;3(6C):3.
7. Nahas SJ. Diagnosis of acute headache. Curr Pain Headache Rep 2011;15:94–7.
8. Yu YE, Schwedt TJ. Abrupt-onset severe headaches. Semin Neurol 2010;30(2): 192–200.

9. Dupont SA, Wijdicks EF, Manno EM, et al. Thunderclap headache and normal computed tomographic results: value of cerebrospinal fluid analysis. Mayo Clin Proc 2008;83(12):1326–31.

10. Horstman P, Linn FH, Voorbij HA, et al. Chance of aneurysm in patients suspected of SAH who have a 'negative' CT scan but a 'positive' lumbar puncture. J Neurol 2012;259(4):649–52.

11. Abend N, Younkin D. Medical causes of headaches in children. Curr Pain Headache Rep 2007;11:401–7.

12. Gladstein J. Secondary headaches. Curr Pain Headache Rep 2006;10:382–6.

13. Ahad R, Kossoff EH. Secondary intracranial causes for headaches in children. Curr Pain Headache Rep 2008;12:373–8.

14. Goldlust SA, Graber JJ, Bossert DF, et al. Headache in patients with cancer. Curr Pain Headache Rep 2010;14:455–64.

15. Gladstone J, Bigal ME. Headaches attributable to infectious diseases. Curr Pain Headache Rep 2010;14:299–308.

16. Loder E, Cardona L. Evaluation for secondary causes of headache: the role of blood and urine testing. Headache 2011;9:341–4.

17. Bigal ME, Gladstone J. The metabolic headaches. Curr Pain Headache Rep 2008;12:292–5.

18. Goffaux P, Fortin D. Brain tumor headaches: from bedside to bench. Neurosurgery 2010;67:459–66.

19. Matthew PG, Garza I. Headache. Semin Neurol 2011;31:5–17.

20. Donnet A, Valade D, Houdart E, et al. Primary cough headache, primary exertional headache, and primary headache associated with sexual activity: a clinical and radiological study. Neuroradiology 2012. [Epub ahead of print].

21. Cardona L, Klein AM. Early postpartum headache: case discussions. Semin Neurol 2011;31:385–91.

22. Foley M. Headaches and migraines. Available at: About.com. Accessed November 5, 2012.

23. Wall M. The headache profile of idiopathic intracranial hypertension. Cephalalgia 1990;10:331–5.

24. Davenport R. Headache. Pract Neurol 2008;8:335–43.

25. Larner AJ. Not all morning headaches are due to brain tumor. Pract Neurol 2009;9:80–4.

26. Pearce JM. Clinical features of the exploding head syndrome. J Neurol Neurosurg Psychiatry 1989;52:907–10.

27. Rinkel GJ, Djibuti M, Algra A, et al. Prevalence and risk of rupture of intracranial aneurysms: a systematic review. Stroke 1998;29(1):251–6.

28. Bederson JB, Connolly ES Jr, Batjer HH, et al. Guidelines for the management of aneurysmal subarachnoid hemorrhage: a statement for healthcare professionals from a special writing group of the Stroke Council, American Heart Association. Stroke 2009;40(3):994–1025.

29. Friedman BW, Lipton RB. Headache emergencies: diagnosis and management. Neurol Clin 2012;30:43–59.

Imaging in the Evaluation of Headache

Malisa S. Lester, MD, Benjamin P. Liu, MD*

KEYWORDS

- Headache • CT • MRI • Imaging • Neuroimaging • Diagnosis • Guidelines

KEY POINTS

- Although most headaches are a primary headache disorder with a benign course, imaging is an important part of the diagnostic evaluation to exclude the presence of a secondary cause of headache that could cause fatal results or severe neurologic morbidity.
- In patients with headache but without focal neurologic examination abnormalities, the yield of neuroimaging for significant intracranial findings is generally low.
- Certain subgroups of patients with headache and headache presentations have high rates of significant intracranial abnormalities, including hemorrhage, infarction, and tumor.
- For headaches that are suspicious for intracranial hemorrhage, particularly those presenting acutely, the initial neuroimaging study is usually a CT scan.
- Headaches presenting with a chronic course or in the outpatient setting can usually be initially studied with MRI.

INTRODUCTION

Headache is an extremely common symptom with a wide differential and can be due to hundreds of causes. Annually, more than 70% of the United States population may have a headache.[1,2] In contrast, the frequency of pathologic conditions that present with headache is rather low and most headaches are due to benign primary headache disorders.[1,3] The overall yield of neuroimaging studies for headache without an abnormality on neurologic examination is low, ranging from 0.5% to 3% in the literature.[3–9] A meta-analysis of retrospective studies of imaging in headache patients from combined inpatient, outpatient, and emergency room settings revealed significant abnormalities in 7.2%.[10] A prospective study of chronic headaches seen in a neurology clinic had a 1.2% rate of significant abnormalities on imaging.[11] However, secondary causes of headache can have devastating consequences or important treatment implications,

Disclosures: None.

Section of Neuroradiology, Department of Radiology, Northwestern Memorial Hospital, Feinberg School of Medicine of Northwestern University, 676 North Saint Clair Street, 14th Floor, Chicago, IL 60611, USA

* Corresponding author.

E-mail address: bliu@nmff.org

Med Clin N Am 97 (2013) 243–265

http://dx.doi.org/10.1016/j.mcna.2012.11.004

0025-7125/13/$ – see front matter © 2013 Elsevier Inc. All rights reserved.

medical.theclinics.com

thus it is important to obtain imaging appropriately to differentiate between secondary and primary headache disorders as defined by the *International Classification of Headache Disorders*, 2nd edition (ICHD-2).[12] This article reviews when and how to use imaging for headaches, and what abnormalities may be found on these studies.

WHEN TO PERFORM IMAGING

Recommendations regarding when to perform imaging for headache have been published by groups such as the US Headache Consortium,[5] American Academy of Neurology,[13] American College of Emergency Physicians (ACEP),[14] and American College of Radiology (ACR).[15] Although these guidelines can serve as a starting point in clinical decision making, these guidelines are not all inclusive, and some are hedged by uncertainties. There are numerous indications that are not covered by consensus or society guidelines. The heterogeneity of the existing evidence contributes to the difficulty of developing comprehensive uniform guidelines.[16] Other investigators and groups have also consolidated or meta-analyzed imaging guidelines.[1,2,4,10,17–19] In the setting of imperfect data and evidence from the literature, clinical judgment and clinician experience play a key role in deciding when to use imaging.

In general, emergent neurologic imaging is recommended for a patient presenting with thunderclap headache with abnormal findings on neurologic examination. Neuroimaging is also generally recommended to determine the safety of lumbar puncture in patients with headache, fever, or nuchal rigidity accompanied by signs of increased intracranial pressure.[2,5,14,18]

The recommendations for when to consider neurologic imaging vary by group; however, several indications are commonly described. Headache features that often warrant neuroimaging include: isolated thunderclap headache, headache radiating to the neck, temporal headache in an older individual, headaches with increasing frequency or severity, headaches always occurring on the same side, and headaches not responding to treatment. Patient demographics that should prompt consideration of imaging are a new headache in a patient who is HIV positive, has a prior history of cancer, is pregnant, has seizures, or is older than 50 years of age. Associated symptoms and signs occurring with headache that may prompt neuroimaging include headache accompanied by abnormal neurologic examination findings (eg, papilledema, unilateral loss of sensation, unilateral weakness, or unilateral hyperreflexia), cognitive impairment, and personality change. Abnormality on neurologic examination is the most consistent and robust predictor of intracranial pathologic conditions on subsequent imaging. Additional conditions in which there has been some reported increased likelihood of intracranial abnormality include headaches that are worsened by Valsalva maneuver, headaches that wake the patient from sleep, and headaches with emesis. Postural headaches and headaches triggered by cough, exertion, or sexual activity have also been described as indications for neuroimaging.[2,3,10,15,17,18]

Many guidelines and literature reviews suggest that neurologic imaging is usually not warranted for a migraine headache with normal neurologic examination findings, although exceptions can exist[20] and clinical judgment is important. Imaging is also usually not warranted when there is no significant change in the pattern of a longstanding headache; no new worrisome features, such as fever, seizure, or trauma; no focal neurologic symptoms or signs; and no high risk factors on clinical presentation.

HOW TO PERFORM IMAGING

The imaging modality, use of intravenous contrast, and the imaging sequences to be obtained are all important parameters when performing imaging. In general, CT is a faster and more readily available modality that should be used in urgent clinical situations. CT is generally preferred to MRI for evaluation of subarachnoid hemorrhage (SAH), acute head trauma, and bone abnormalities. On the other hand, MRI is considered superior to CT for evaluation of the brain parenchyma and soft tissue structures. MRI is generally preferred for evaluation of cerebral infarctions, intracranial neoplasm, intracranial infection, and other forms of intracranial pathologic conditions, such as Chiari malformation, intracranial hypotension, pituitary lesions, and encephalopathies. CT angiography (CTA) and MR angiography (MRA), as well as CT venography (CTV) and MR venography (MRV), are available for evaluation of vascular lesions in addition to conventional catheter angiography. An important feature of CT imaging to keep in mind is the associated radiation exposure. In the end, choosing the imaging modality and protocol should be directed by clinical suspicion and in consultation with a radiologist specializing in neuroimaging.

In the acute setting, a general algorithm for neuroimaging would be an emergent non–contrast CT head scan for patients presenting with the worst headache of life or sudden severe thunderclap headache. If there is evidence of SAH or a mass lesion, further neuroimaging would be warranted depending on the underlying lesion suspected. Neurosurgical consultation is often needed in these diagnoses. Other intracranial hemorrhages, including epidural, subdural, and parenchymal, also often require neurosurgical consultation. If the CT does not demonstrate a finding to explain the patient's headache, an MRI of the head should be considered. Additional tests, such as CTA, MRA, or lumbar puncture, may also be considered.

For patients presenting with other indications to obtain neuroimaging, and when acute intracranial hemorrhage is thought to be less likely clinically, a CT scan is recommended only for urgent clinical indications or when MRI is not available (eg, to exclude midline shift before lumbar puncture or to evaluate for hydrocephalus). Otherwise, MRI is the preferred modality and consultation with a radiologist is suggested to optimize the imaging protocol. Optimal MRI evaluation of inflammatory, infectious, neoplastic, and demyelinating conditions uses intravenous contrast in patients with appropriate renal function. Gradient-echo (GRE) sequences can be helpful for evaluation of intracranial hemorrhage although CT is still the preferred first-line modality for imaging of acute intracranial hemorrhage. Fluid-attenuated inversion recovery (FLAIR) sequences are useful for evaluation of cerebral edema and occasionally detects subtle SAH, and diffusion-weighted imaging (DWI) sequences are necessary if acute infarction is of clinical concern. Advanced MRI techniques, such as MR spectroscopy (MRS) or MR perfusion, can help characterize neoplastic masses and differentiate them from nonneoplastic entities. Fat-suppressed T1-weighted images are useful in the evaluation of vascular dissection.

WHAT ABNORMALITIES MAY BE FOUND

When a specific diagnosis is suspected, a distinctive presentation occurs, or a particular population is being evaluated, a focused imaging strategy can be tailored to the case. **Box 1** highlights groups of headache patients and headache presentations with high rates of intracranial abnormality on imaging. An in-depth discussion of specific diagnoses, populations, and headache presentations follows.

Subarachnoid Hemorrhage

The most worrisome presentation of headache is the sudden onset, severe thunderclap headache. When a patient presents with a thunderclap headache, conservative estimates of finding SAH is in the range of 11% to 25%[14,17] but may be up to

> **Box 1**
> **Groups of headache patients and headache presentations with high rates of significant intracranial abnormality on imaging**
>
> 1. Thunderclap headache presentations had acute SAH at conservatively estimated rates of 11% to 25% but may be as high as 47%.
>
> 2. Approximately one-third of patients with cancer presenting with a new or changed headache will have intracranial metastases.
>
> 3. Approximately one-fourth of pregnant patients presenting with acute headache to the emergency department had a significant cause to explain their headache found on neuroimaging.
>
> 4. Up to 30% of trauma patients with a normal neurologic examination may have associated intracranial abnormality.
>
> 5. HIV-positive patients had between 35% and 82% yield of intracranial abnormalities on neuroimaging studies.

47%.[3,10] Although SAH is the most often considered diagnosis for thunderclap headache, there are other causes of this headache presentation. The conventional algorithm for evaluation of SAH is a non–contrast head CT that, if negative, is followed by a lumbar puncture. A non–contrast head CT is 92% to 95% sensitive for detection of acute SAH on the day of the aneurysm rupture but decreases in sensitivity on subsequent days.[14,17] The sensitivity of CT for detection of SAH is limited by numerous factors, including the inability of scanners to identify small hemorrhages in areas obscured by artifact or bone, interreader variability, spectrum bias in small-volume SAH, decreased sensitivity for blood in the setting of anemia, and decay in sensitivity with time.[14] Performing a lumbar puncture after a negative CT increases the diagnostic certainty. Estimates of rates of SAH confirmed by lumbar puncture after negative CT results are in the range of 2.5% to 3.5%.[14] Timing is also an important factor affecting lumbar puncture in detecting SAH. The sensitivity for detecting xanthochromia is also subject to decay the more days or weeks pass after initial SAH. In addition, if lumbar puncture is performed too soon, within 12 hours of bleeding, it may be falsely negative. If SAH is detected on CT or lumbar puncture, angiographic imaging should be performed to determine if there is an aneurysm (**Fig. 1**). CTA or MRA can be performed depending on institutional preference. The workup will likely also include conventional catheter cerebral angiography. If no aneurysms are detected after adequate and satisfactory angiographic imaging, the diagnosis of exclusion in atraumatic subarachnoid bleeding is benign perimesencephalic bleeding that tends to have a benign course. Repeat neuroimaging to diagnose intracranial hemorrhage when initial results are equivocal and early imaging when there is high suspicion for intracranial hemorrhage are both clinically prudent. Changing the diagnostic paradigm for SAH after a negative CT to CTA instead of lumbar puncture is controversial[21] and based in part on the notion that expansion or thrombosis of an unruptured intracranial aneurysm may be a cause of headache.

Other Intracranial Bleeding

Other intracranial hemorrhages that may present with headache include subdural hematoma (SDH), epidural hematoma, and parenchymal hemorrhage. SDHs are often seen in the elderly and may present after relatively minor head trauma or subacute to remote trauma (**Fig. 2**). Conversely, epidural hematomas often occur after high-energy trauma and are caused by a blow to the squamosal temporal bone with injury of the

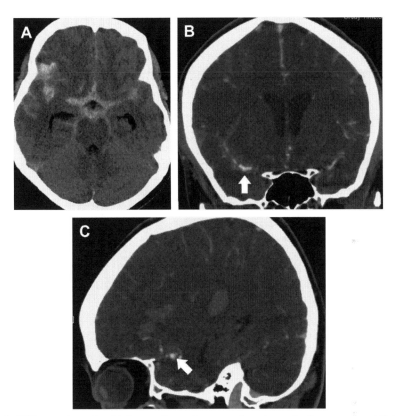

Fig. 1. Diffuse subarachnoid hemorrhage from ruptured cerebral aneurysm. (*A*) Non–contrast-enhanced CT of hyperdense acute SAH throughout the suprasellar cistern and within the right sylvian fissure. (*B*) Coronal CTA image of a complex, multilobulated aneurysm at the right middle cerebral artery (MCA) bifurcation (*arrow*). SAH within the right sylvian fissure is more difficult to appreciate on the postcontrast CTA images but is present. (*C*) Sagittal CTA image of a complex, multilobulated aneurysm at the right MCA bifurcation (*arrow*). SAH, subarachnoid hemorrhage.

middle meningeal artery (**Fig. 3**). Parenchymal bleeding may be due to hemorrhagic metastasis, cerebral amyloid angiopathy (CAA), arterial venous malformation, other underlying vascular anomaly, or coagulopathy (**Fig. 4**).

Arteriovenous malformations (AVMs) are 10 times less common then aneurysms and only a fraction of them present with isolated headache.[3] They can present with either acute parenchymal or subarachnoid bleeding. AVMs can be characterized using CTA or MRI and/or MRA but are best characterized by conventional cerebral angiography (**Fig. 5**). Presence of associated intranidal or feeding artery aneurysms increases the risk of AVM hemorrhage.

Cavernous malformations account for 10% to 15% of intracranial and spinal vascular malformations and are made up of a compact mass of sinusoidal-type vessels without normal intervening brain. On CT these are usually hyperdense and on MRI are well circumscribed masses with a rim of T2 hypointensity and marked gradient susceptibility signal (**Fig. 6**). When these lesions bleed, they may increase in size on imaging, become associated with vasogenic edema, or show acute hemorrhage.

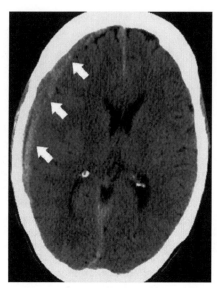

Fig. 2. SDH. NECT image of a mildly hyperdense acute right cerebral hemispheric SDH (*arrows*) associated with local mass effect, local sulcal effacement, and slight leftward midline shift. SDH, subdural hematoma; NECT, noncontrast head CT.

A significant association exists between CAA and lobar intracerebral hemorrhage (ICH).[22] If the diagnosis has not been established pathologically via brain biopsy, probable and possible diagnoses of CAA can be made by imaging, according to the Boston criteria.[23] MRI is more sensitive for presence of disease compared with CT, whereas CT can better evaluate acute bleeding. In patients greater than age 60, when MRI demonstrates multifocal peripheral lobar sites of gradient susceptibility on the GRE

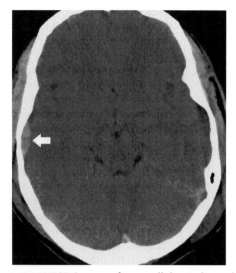

Fig. 3. Epidural hematoma. NECT image of a small hyperdense lentiform acute right temporal epidural hematoma (*arrow*).

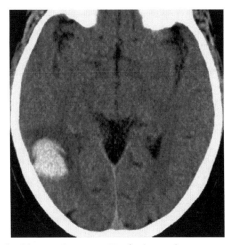

Fig. 4. Lobar intracerebral hemorrhage. NECT of a hyperdense acute right temporoparietal parenchymal hematoma, associated with local mass effect and local sulcal effacement. Low attenuation surrounding the hematoma is compatible with associated surrounding edema.

MRI sequence, the diagnosis of CAA is suspected. CAA may be found diffusely in the brain, or localized to one lobe or hemisphere.

Anticoagulation and Coagulopathy

Conventional intensities of oral anticoagulation increase the rate of intracranial bleeding 7-fold to 10-fold, to an absolute rate of nearly 1% per year for many stroke-prone patients. Aspirin seems to double the risk for ICH, regardless of the dose. Most are ICH (70%), whereas most of the rest are SDH. Predictors of anticoagulant-related ICH are advanced patient age, prior ischemic stroke,

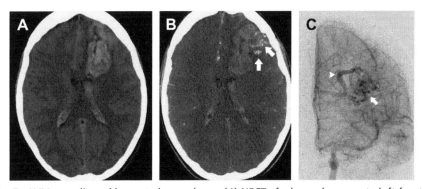

Fig. 5. AVM complicated by acute hemorrhage. (*A*) NECT of a hyperdense acute left frontal lobe parenchymal hematoma with intraventricular extension and some associated local SAH. (*B*) CTA image of an adjacent cluster of prominent vessels in the left frontal lobe (*arrows*), suspicious for an AVM. (*C*) Conventional cerebral angiography image during injection of the left internal carotid artery of an abnormal nidus of vessels in the left frontal lobe (*arrow*) associated with a large draining vein (*arrowhead*), confirming the presence of an AVM. AVM, arteriovenous malformation.

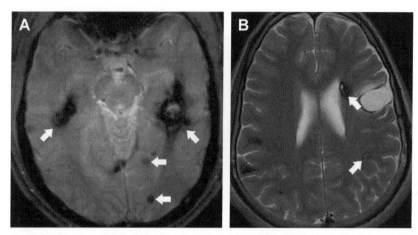

Fig. 6. Multiple cavernomas. (*A*) Axial GRE MRI of multiple foci of gradient susceptibility blooming (*arrows*) in the bilateral temporal and left occipital lobes. (*B*) Axial T2-weighted MRI, in the same patient at a different level, of multiple foci of round hyperintense T2 signal with a rim of hypointense T2 signal (*arrows*, representative lesions), compatible with multiple cavernomas. GRE, gradient echo.

hypertension, minor trauma, and intensity of anticoagulation. Acute intracranial hemorrhages are well identified on noncontrast head CT, and in anticoagulated patients, an almost unique fluid-blood interface in the ICH may be seen within the first 12 hours as a result of uncongealed blood. Symptoms, including the onset of unusual headache, nausea and vomiting, confusion, ataxia, or dizziness, in elderly patients on oral anticoagulants should prompt urgent evaluation for intracranial hemorrhage.[24] Substantially lower rates of intracranial hemorrhage and traumatic intracranial bleeds were seen in elderly atrial fibrillation patients receiving dabigatran (Pradaxa) compared with warfarin (Coumadin).[25] Neuroimaging is also important for evaluating intracranial hemorrhage in patients with coagulopathies such as hemophilia[26] and leukemia with thrombocytopenia.[27]

Tumor

The annual incidence of intracranial tumor is extremely low. In the United States, it was approximately 30 per 100,000 from 2006 to 2010.[28] In the United Kingdom, the incidence ranges between 10 and 60 per 100,000.[29] Are there clinical symptoms or signs that indicate a particular level of risk of finding intracranial tumor to help guide when to perform neuroimaging? One group of investigators suggested three levels of risk stratification based on evaluation of existing evidence and expert clinical opinion.[29] Urgent investigation was suggested for presentations in which the risk of finding intracranial tumor was greater than 1%. These presentations include headache with a history of known cancer elsewhere; headache with abnormal neurologic examination; evidence of increased intracranial pressure; significant alterations in consciousness, memory, confusion, or coordination; and new epileptic seizure. Of patients with cancer presenting with new or changed headache, 32% will have intracranial metastases. Cluster headaches were also considered in this category. In the next category where the probability of finding intracranial tumor was between 0.1% and 1%, careful monitoring and a low threshold for investigation were suggested. These presentations included new headache in which a diagnostic pattern has not emerged after 8 weeks from presentation; headache with abnormal neurologic symptoms, such as those aggravated by exertion or Valsalva; headache with vomiting; significant changes in characteristics of chronic headaches, such as rapid increase in frequency; new headache in a patient over 50 years; headaches that awake the patient from sleep; and confusion. In the last category, in which the probability of finding intracranial tumor was less than 0.1% but still above the background population incidence, appropriate management was suggested and the need for follow-up not excluded. Presentations in this group included diagnosis of migraine or tension-type headache, weakness or motor loss, memory loss, and personality change.

In general, MRI is more sensitive than CT for detection of intracranial tumor (**Fig. 7**). Specialized MRI sequences are preferable to assess for tumor in the sellar, cerebello-pontine angle, and internal auditory canal regions. Findings may include intracranial mass, leptomeningeal or dural disease, and osseous tumor; as well as secondary complications, including intracranial mass effect, edema, herniation, hemorrhage, or hydrocephalus. Significant osseous, extracranial soft tissue, or cervical soft tissue involvement by tumor can cause pain resembling headache. Although CT is generally considered better than MRI for assessing bone tumor, detection of osseous tumor and any associated paraosseous involvement in the calvarium, skull base, or cervical spine may require a combination of radiographs, CT, MRI, bone scan, positron emission tomography (PET)-CT, or other studies depending on the individual scenario. Bone scan has the benefit of surveying for osseous tumor elsewhere in the body. PET-CT also scans a large portion of the body and helps in identification of the site of an unknown primary.

Hydrocephalus and Increased Intracranial Pressure

On imaging, communicating hydrocephalus shows enlargement of the lateral, third, and fourth ventricles. This is often due to impairment of cerebrospinal fluid (CSF) reab-sorption at the level of the arachnoid granulations, which can be due to remote SAH or

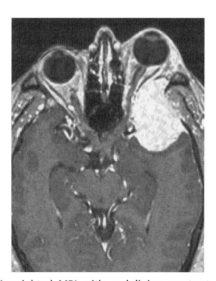

Fig. 7. Tumor. Axial T1-weighted MRI with gadolinium contrast of an enhancing mass centered at the left sphenoid bone, causing mass effect on the anterior left temporal lobe, spreading into the left orbit with resulting left sided proptosis, and eroding the under-lying sphenoid bone. The pathologic condition of this mass was plasmacytoma; patient later went on to develop multiple myeloma.

intracranial infection. Obstructive hydrocephalus has different imaging presentations depending on the site of obstruction. Unilateral enlargement of a lateral ventricle may occur from obstruction at the level of the foramen of Monroe (ie, colloid cyst or intraventricular tumor) or local trapping within the lateral ventricle (ie, scar tissue). Triventricular enlargement of the lateral and third ventricles can occur from obstruction at the level of the cerebral aqueduct, such as from aqueductal stenosis, pineal mass, or tectal mass. Clinical symptoms of hydrocephalus include headache, memory impairment, gait unsteadiness and falls, and visual disturbances related to papilledema.[30]

Patients with clinical signs of increased intracranial pressure (eg, papilledema, absent venous pulsations on funduscopic examination, altered mental status, focal neurologic deficits, or signs of meningeal irritation) should have neuroimaging before a lumbar puncture.[14] Imaging signs of increased intracranial pressure include midline shift, effacement of cerebral sulci from diffuse cerebral edema, and herniation. Several forms of herniation exist, including subfalcine herniation, transtentorial herniation, uncal herniation, and cerebellar tonsillar herniation.

Infarction

Headaches associated with acute stroke are frequent, and often resemble a reactivation of the patient's previous headaches pattern.[31] The International Headache Society reports that headache accompanies ischemic stroke in 17% to 34% of cases.[12] Similar ranges were reported in other observational studies (**Fig. 8**).[32,33] Acute infarctions related to dissection are also associated with headache. The association of headaches at stroke onset is seen in younger patient and those with a history of migraine. In addition, headaches related to stroke are usually vertebrobasilar strokes, rather than anterior circulation strokes, and are usually cerebellar strokes.[34] When there is concern for acute ischemic infarction associated with headache, MRI with DWI needs to be obtained.

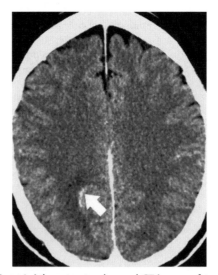

Fig. 8. Cerebral infarction. Axial contrast-enhanced CT image of typical mild enhancement at the edge of a subacute stroke in the right parietal lobe (*arrow*). Adjacent areas of low attenuation represent resolving edema and early gliosis. The patient had a new headache since open heart surgery several weeks ago due to a perioperative stroke.

Migrainous infarction occurs in a very small subset of migraine patients, and the rate is about 0.8 per 100,000 person-year. Although this is less than 1% of all ischemic strokes, it may account for up to 20% of ischemic strokes in the younger population.[35] Migraine with aura is a risk factor for ischemic stroke in women under age 45 years, particularly when combined with other risk factors such as smoking and oral contraceptives.[35] According to ICHD-2, migrainous infarction is a typical attack of migrainous aura in a patient with previous history of migraines with aura and ischemic stroke proven by neuroimaging. If a concomitant cause is detected (eg, dissection, cardiac arrhythmia, coagulopathy, or paradoxic embolism in presence of a patent foramen ovale) or if a patient with a history of migraines without aura develops ischemic stroke after a migraine attack, the disease is not considered migrainous infarction but instead ischemic stroke coexisting with migraine.[35,36]

Cerebral autosomal dominant arteriopathy with subcortical infarcts and leukoencephalopathy (CADASIL) is a rare encephalopathy seen in adults with recurrent headaches; however, is the most common form of hereditary stroke disorder. These patients present with recurrent strokes associated with headaches and are diagnosed by genetic testing. MRI reveals numerous and usually extensive chronic infarcts throughout the cerebral white matter, and there is distinctive involvement in the anterior temporal lobes that, in contrast, is atypical for chronic small vessel white matter ischemic disease from chronic hypertensive encephalopathy.

Vascular Abnormalities

Dissection
A new onset headache, usually unilateral, that is radiating into the neck should be concerning for dissection. Symptoms may include ipsilateral Horner syndrome. Given the appropriate clinical history, this can be diagnosed using CTA or MRA. If MRA is performed, the T1 axial fat-saturated sequence is routinely added for evaluation of intramural hematoma. The presence of T1 hyperintense intramural hematoma is seen in dissections between 1 week to 8 weeks of age (**Fig. 9**). At 6 months, intramural T1

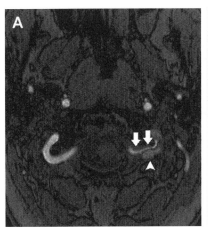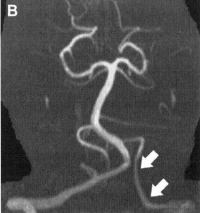

Fig. 9. Dissection. (*A*) Axial MRA image of an asymmetrically irregular and stenotic distal V3 segment of the left vertebral artery (*arrows*) surrounded by intrinsic T1 hyperintense signal (*arrowhead*), compatible with an acute left vertebral artery dissection and associated intramural hematoma. (*B*) Maximum-intensity-projection (MIP) reconstructed image from the MRA of asymmetric stenosis and irregularity (*arrows*) consistent with acute distal left vertebral artery dissection.

hyperintensity will have resolved.[37] MRI with DWI should also be considered to evaluate for any associated strokes.

Cerebral venous thrombosis
Increased risk of cerebral venous thrombosis (CVT) is seen in the postpartum period, hypercoagulable disorders; increased hematocrit states; severe dehydration; local infection adjacent to a dural sinus, such as mastoiditis; and after trauma. Dural venous thrombosis or cortical venous thrombosis can be characterized by CTV or MRV **(Fig. 10)**. Prolonged or extensive CVT may result in a venous infarction, for which MRI with DWI should be considered.

Giant cell arteritis
In an elderly patient presenting with temporal headaches and elevated sedimentation rate, giant cell arteritis should be suspected.[38] This is primarily a clinical and laboratory diagnosis and, although it is mainly a vasculitis of large and medium vessels that classically involves the external carotid artery branches (ie, the superficial temporal artery), there exists a rare risk of intracranial vasculitis. Although uncommon, intracranial vasculitis can result in brainstem strokes.[39,40] Urgent treatment with steroids may prevent vision loss or brainstem strokes. A non–contrast CT is necessary as the initial study in the evaluation of stroke; however, it may miss brainstem and cerebellar infarcts due to the technical limitations of CT. When there is a high degree of clinical suspicion, MRI or MRA head scans should be obtained to rule out acute stroke in the posterior fossa or identify evidence of vasculitis **(Fig. 11)**.

Reversible cerebral vasoconstriction syndrome
Reversible cerebral vasoconstriction syndrome (RCVS) is characterized by the association of severe headaches with or without additional neurologic symptoms and a vasospasmed or string-and-beads appearance of the medium and small intracranial arteries

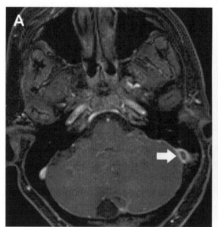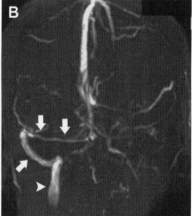

Fig. 10. CVT. (*A*) Axial image from an MRV with gadolinium contrast of a filling defect, compatible with thrombus, in the left sigmoid sinus (*arrow*). (*B*) MIP image from an MRV without gadolinium contrast of an asymmetric lack of flow signal in the left transverse and sigmoid sinus, as well as the proximal left internal jugular vein, compatible with the presence of venous sinus thrombosis. The right transverse and sigmoid sinuses (*arrows*), right internal jugular vein (*arrowhead*), and the superior sagittal sinus show expected flow signal. CVT, cerebral venous thrombosis; MRV, magnetic resonance venography; MIP, maximum intensity projection.

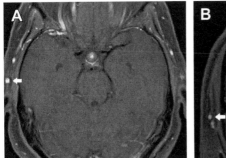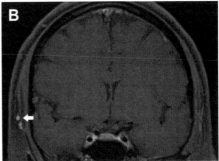

Fig. 11. Giant cell arteritis. (*A*) Axial T1-weighted postcontrast fat-saturated MRI of asymmetric thickening and enhancement of the right superficial temporal artery walls (*arrow*). There was no imaging evidence of intracranial vasculitis. (*B*) Coronal T1-weighted postcontrast fat-saturated MRI of asymmetric thickening and enhancement of the right superficial temporal artery walls (*arrow*). There was no imaging evidence of intracranial vasculitis.

that resolves spontaneously in 1 to 3 months. Recent severe headache was, by definition, the presenting symptom of the patients in one case series.[41] Recurrent thunderclap headaches, seizures, strokes, and nonaneurysmal SAH can all be associated with RCVS. The syndrome may be spontaneous and idiopathic, or it may be secondary to various causes, including postpartum period and exposure to vasoactive substances such as cannabis, selective serotonin reuptake inhibitors, and nasal decongestants. The course is typically benign and supportive treatment is recommended. MRA, CTA, or conventional cerebral angiography may be used to diagnose this condition.[41,42]

Moyamoya disease
Moyamoya is an uncommon disease characterized by stenosis or occlusion of the distal internal carotid arteries and their branches. Collateral lenticulostriate vessels develop in an attempt to compensate for the decreased blood flow in the anterior circulation and produce the namesake characteristic puff of smoke appearance of this disease on angiography. Headache associated with moyamoya disease is common and can persist even after successful surgical revascularization. Aneurysms and AVMs are frequently associated in 11% to 14% of cases.[43]

Pregnancy and Postpartum Period

Patients presenting with headache during pregnancy or postpartum period seem to have a higher yield of intracranial pathologic conditions than the general population and require careful consideration for imaging. In one study, neuroimaging, including non–contrast head CT and MRI, revealed an underlying headache cause in 27% of pregnant patients presenting to an emergency department. Diagnoses included CVT, posterior reversible encephalopathy syndrome (PRES), pseudotumor, and intracranial hemorrhage. The odds of having an intracranial abnormality on neuroimaging were 2.7 times higher in patients with an abnormal neurologic examination.[44]

Several secondary causes of headache are unique to pregnancy and the postpartum period, whereas others are of increased incidence. A pregnant patient is 5 times more likely to develop SAH than a nonpregnant patient. The risk of infarction is markedly increased in the first few weeks postpartum. Risk of CVT is greatest in the first 2 to 4 weeks following delivery. During preeclampsia or eclampsia patients can present clinically with hypertensive encephalopathy, identical to findings seen with PRES (**Fig. 12**). Postpartum angiopathy is considered by some to be in the

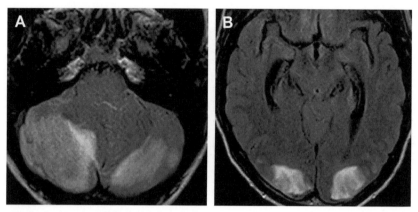

Fig. 12. Posterior reversible leukoencephalopathy syndrome. (*A*) Axial FLAIR MRI of relatively symmetric areas of hyperintense FLAIR signal in the posterior bilateral cerebellar hemispheres with associated edema and swelling. (*B*) Axial FLAIR MRI in the same patient of a higher level relatively symmetric areas of hyperintense FLAIR signal in the posterior bilateral occipital lobes. Given the posterior distribution, this was consistent with PRES. PRES, posterior reversible leukoencephalopathy syndrome; FLAIR, fluid attenuation inversion recovery.

same spectrum as RCVS and shares similarities with eclampsia and PRES on imaging. Amniotic fluid embolism to the intracranial vasculature resembles embolic strokes given involvement of multiple vascular territories by restricted diffusion and associated vasogenic edema. Several pregnancy-related malignancies exist ranging from benign hydatidiform molar to invasive molar pregnancy, with the most aggressive subset being choriocarcinoma. Choriocarcinoma metastases to the brain are often hemorrhagic. The hormonal changes of pregnancy may cause a trophic effect on some central nervous system neoplasms, including meningiomas, ependymomas, hemangioblastomas, pituitary adenomas, and schwannomas; as well as metastases, such as melanoma or breast carcinoma. Sheehan syndrome is pituitary hypothalamic dysfunction related to pituitary ischemia and necrosis. Pituitary apoplexy describes an acute hemorrhagic infarction of the pituitary gland, commonly in a preexisting adenoma (**Fig. 13**). Postdural puncture headaches are a consideration in the postpartum period.[44,45]

During pregnancy, special considerations for imaging include radiation dose and contrast administration. The ACR and the American College of Obstetricians and Gynecologists have provided similar guidance in this area. A radiation-protection paradigm that has been promoted that emphasizes lowering radiation as much as possible is a principle known as ALARA (As Low As Reasonably Achievable).[45] In practice, at the most conservative level, fetal doses of less than 5 rad have not been associated with an increase in fetal anomaly or pregnancy loss. Fetal dose associated with a head CT is considered to be less than 0.01 rad. A non–contrast CT head scan is useful to rule out life-threatening conditions such as subarachnoid or parenchymal hemorrhage.

If MRI is used, there is no radiation dose. An MRI brain scan without gadolinium is safe in all trimesters in pregnancy and, in fact, is the preferred imaging modality to search for structural causes of secondary headaches in pregnancy. No current evidence exists that would suggest harm to the fetus exposed to magnetic fields up to 3 T. Most intracranial abnormalities during pregnancy can be diagnosed using non–contrast MRI techniques, but contrast is useful for select indications and can be administered if the benefits outweigh the risks.[17,19,45]

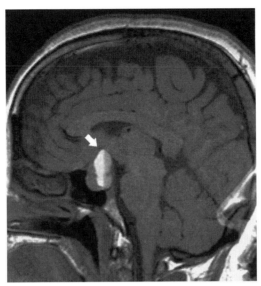

Fig. 13. Pituitary apoplexy. Sagittal T1-weighted MRI of T1 hyperintense hemorrhage in a pituitary macroadenoma. A blood-fluid level can be seen in the hemorrhage because patient is supine on the MRI scanner table. Superior extension of the mass into the suprasellar cistern causes mass effect on the optic chiasm (*arrow*). Clinically, this patient presented with headache and bitemporal hemianopia.

Intravenous administration of iodinated contrast for CT to the pregnant patient has not been associated with any teratogenic effect. However, some studies have raised concerns for neonatal hypothyroidism. Therefore, intravenous iodinated contrast administration should be deferred during pregnancy when possible. For examinations, such as CTV or CTA, for which contrast is required, it can be administered with subsequent hypothyroidism screening of the infant in the neonatal period. The administration of gadolinium-based MRI contrast should be deferred during pregnancy when possible but may be administered if clinically necessary because no risk has been specifically found.

If a lactating patient receives intravenous iodinated or gadolinium-based contrast, discarding breast milk (pump and dump) may be recommended for 24 hours after contrast administration.[45]

Pediatric Headaches

Similar to adult literature, studies in the pediatric population show a low likelihood of finding a significant intracranial abnormality in children with headaches and normal neurologic examinations.[1] The current recommendations by the Quality Standards Subcommittee of the American Academy of Neurology and the Practice Committee of the Child Neurology Society are that obtaining a neuroimaging study on a routine basis is not indicated in children with recurrent headaches and a normal neurologic examination.[46] They recommend that neuroimaging be considered in children with an abnormal neurologic examination (eg, focal findings, signs of increased intracranial pressure, or significant alteration of consciousness), the coexistence of seizures, or both. Additionally, they recommend consideration of neuroimaging in children in whom there are historical features to suggest the recent onset of severe headache, there is a change in the type of headache, or who have associated features that suggest neurologic dysfunction (eg, headache associated with substantial episodes of confusion, disorientation, or emesis).

Other indications in the literature for considering neuroimaging in children with headaches include persistent headaches of less than 6-months duration that do not respond to medical treatment, persistent headache associated with an absent family history of migraine, and headaches that awaken a child repeatedly from sleep or occur immediately on awakening. Presence of a ventriculoperitoneal shunt may require imaging to evaluate for shunt dysfunction. A family history or medical history of disorders that may predispose a child to central nervous system lesions and clinical or laboratory findings that also suggest central nervous system involvement may warrant consideration of neuroimaging.[19]

Infection and Immunosuppression

Often, lumbar puncture will be indicated in cases of suspected meningitis and encephalitis. Patients with clinical signs of increased intracranial pressure should have neuroimaging before a lumbar puncture.[14] The extent of encephalitis and response to treatment is best evaluated using MRI with contrast (**Fig. 14**). Parenchymal hemorrhage is common in some infections, such as herpes encephalitis, and can be identified on CT or MRI. Brain abscess is best characterized on MRI with DWI as a cystic or necrotic mass with usually homogeneous restricted diffusion. Endocarditis may lead to multiple intracranial complications, including septic embolic infarcts which may be associated with hemorrhage and mycotic aneurysms.

Immunocompromised patients due to HIV, malignancies, or medical immunosuppression are at risk for opportunistic intracranial infections. HIV-positive patients presenting with a new type of headache should be considered for an urgent neuroimaging

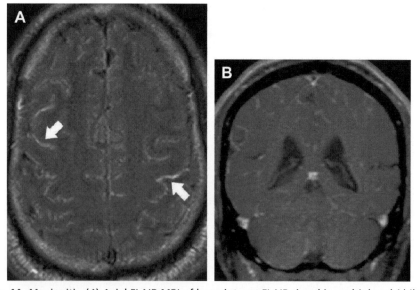

Fig. 14. Meningitis. (A) Axial FLAIR MRI of hyperintense FLAIR signal in multiple sulci bilaterally (*arrows*), which can be seen in the setting of meningitis or SAH, among other differential diagnoses. (B) Coronal T1-weighted postcontrast fat-saturated MRI of diffuse bilateral sulcal and leptomeningeal enhancement, making this case compatible with meningitis. No imaging evidence of associated encephalitis is identified. FLAIR, fluid attenuation inversion recovery; SAH, subarachnoid hemorrhage.

study.[14,15] HIV-positive patients with headache had a yield of 35% on neuroimaging,[14] but it may be as high as 82%.[3] If a ring-enhancing brain mass is identified in an HIV-positive patient, the differential diagnosis often centers on toxoplasmosis or lymphoma. The distinction can be made using sequential thallium and gallium scintigraphy nuclear medicine studies.[47]

Low Pressure Headaches

Orthostatic or postural headaches may indicate presence of a low pressure headache. Other symptoms can include nonorthostatic headache patterns, visual or aural changes, meningismus, cranial nerve dysfunction, nausea and vomiting, mental status changes, and coma.[48] A recent history of lumbar puncture may be elicited, identifying this as a postdural puncture headache. In other cases, there may be a history of spinal trauma with dural injury or surgical dural tear resulting in CSF leak. Without this history, the headache is often considered spontaneous intracranial hypotension and a site of atraumatic CSF leak may be found on imaging. Spontaneous or idiopathic low pressure headaches are diagnosed by a low opening pressure of less than 6 cm of water according to ICHD-2. Contrast-enhanced brain MRI is much better than CT for the detection of intracranial hypotension. On MRI, findings include bifrontal subdural fluid collections, diffuse dural enhancement and engorgement, and sagging of the brainstem. An acquired Chiari malformation may occur due to sagging (**Fig. 15**). In the spine, diffuse dural enhancement and engorgement of the venous vascular plexus may also be seen. During a search for CSF leak using MRI of the spine, an epidural fluid collection may be identified and is usually found in the cervicothoracic spine in the cases of spontaneous CSF leak, near the surgical site in cases of iatrogenic dural tear (**Fig. 16**), or adjacent to a traumatic dural tear. CSF leaks may also be detected at the skull base after surgery, trauma, or infection. A CSF leak may not be found in all cases, but imaging is clinically directed based on the suspected site of leak.

CT and MR myelography can be used in identifying a spinal CSF leak and locating the site for targeted therapy.[49,50] Radioisotope scintigraphy is a nuclear medicine study that can be used to identify a CSF leak either in the spine or at the skull base. CT and MR myelography are better for the assessment of rapid CSF leaks, whereas scintigraphy may be helpful for the detection of relatively slower leaks. Dynamic CT myelography and digital subtraction myelography are newer techniques for locating

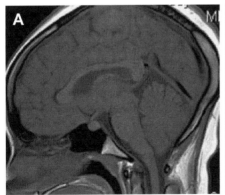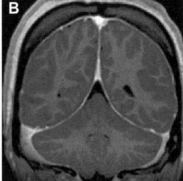

Fig. 15. Spontaneous intracranial hypotension. (*A*) Sagittal T1-weighted MRI of mild sagging of the brain stem and cerebellar tonsils. (*B*) Coronal T1-weighted postcontrast MRI of diffuse, smooth dural thickening and enhancement due to intracranial hypotension.

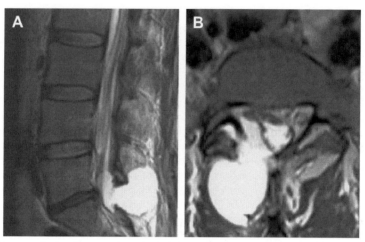

Fig. 16. Iatrogenic dural tear and CSF leak. (A) Sagittal T2-weighted MRI of a large T2 hyperintense epidural and paraspinal fluid collection at the right L5-S1 hemilaminectomy site. (B) Axial T2-weighted MRI of a large T2 hyperintense epidural and paraspinal fluid collection at the right L5-S1 hemilaminectomy site. CSF, cerebrospinal fluid.

the site of very rapid CSF leaks.[51,52] If there is rhinorrhea or otorrhea, pledgets may be placed in the nasal cavities or ears during radioisotope scintigraphy to assess whether the fluid contains CSF leaking radiotracer activity. A CSF leak at the skull base or calvarium can also be characterized by non–contrast CT of the area of interest in the skull base such as paranasal sinuses or temporal bones, by MRI with specialized coronal T2 sequences through the areas of interest, or by CT cisternography using myelographic contrast.

Headaches Associated with Sexual Activity, Exertion, or Coughing

Headaches associated with sexual activity may be a primary or secondary headache disorder. Evidence exists in the literature that some cases of aneurismal SAH are precipitated by sexual intercourse or other forms of intense physical exertion. It is estimated that these activities increase the risk of aneurysm rupture by up to 15-fold.[17,53] In addition, recent literature suggests that intracranial vascular disorders, usually RCVS, are common in this headache type and thus warrant angiographic imaging.[54,55]

When headaches associated with sexual activity present for the first time and the patient is seen very soon after onset, within 48 hours, a non–contrast CT head and a lumbar puncture are suggested to exclude SAH.[17,55,56] Presence of SAH would lead to an appropriate workup of aneurysm, usually including conventional cerebral angiography. If no acute bleed is detected, MRA or CTA of the intracranial and cervical vessels should be obtained. If days or weeks have elapsed since the onset of headaches associated with sexual activity, a contrast-enhanced MRI brain and MRA or CTA of the intracranial and cervical vessels is appropriate.[17]

Secondary exertional headaches may be due to SAH or dissection, which should be excluded by neuroimaging at the first occurrence of these types of headaches.

Secondary causes of headaches associated with Valsalva or cough can include hindbrain malformation or mass lesion, occipitocervical junction disorder, or increased intracranial pressure. The most common finding is a Chiari malformation.[17] Neuroimaging using MRI is most optimal for evaluation of this type of headache and should include sagittal imaging of the occipitocervical junction. If a Chiari malformation is found, cine phase-contrast analysis of CSF flow may reveal restriction of the CSF flow at the level of the foramen magnum and spinal MRI may be necessary to search for any associated syringohydromyelia (**Fig. 17**).

Trauma

Up to 30% of trauma patients with a normal neurologic examination may have associated intracranial abnormality.[17] It is generally accepted that patients identified as having moderate or high risk for intracranial injury should undergo early posttrauma non–contrast CT to rule out ICH, midline shift, or increased intracranial pressure.[57] Intracranial hemorrhages may take time to develop after the initial trauma and, therefore, repeat imaging should be considered for patients with evolving clinical symptoms, worsening headache, or change in headache after trauma and normal initial imaging, particularly within the first 72 hours. Guidelines for imaging after head trauma exist from the ACR and ACEP.[57,58]

Headaches of Orbit, Ear, Nose, and Throat Origin

A variety of disorders in the facial region can also present with headache-like pain or cranial nerve neuralgias, and specific imaging protocols can be used to study the area of interest. These specialized protocols can image the orbits, paranasal sinuses, temporal mandibular joints, specific cranial nerves, temporal bones, or other areas with a higher spatial resolution and a more focused field-of-view than a routine CT or MRI of the head. If there is sinusitis or mastoiditis with suspected intracranial complication of infection such as meningitis or intracranial abscess, the ACR guidelines recommend neuroimaging, usually MRI with contrast, to exclude the intracranial spread of infection. Otherwise, imaging evaluation of sinusitis and mastoiditis can be performed with CT. Reactivation of herpes zoster in the geniculate ganglion can result in Ramsay Hunt syndrome, which can be evaluated using MRI with contrast focusing on the facial nerve course. Temporal mandibular joint dysfunction can be evaluated using CT or MRI, and performing the imaging in open-mouth and closed-mouth configurations is

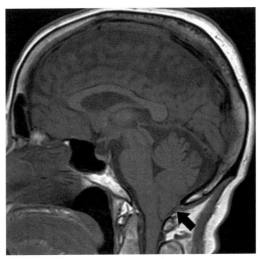

Fig. 17. Chiari malformation. Sagittal T1-weighted MRI of descent of the cerebellar tonsils more than 5 mm below the level of the foramen magnum, with associated crowding at the foramen magnum (*arrow*).

helpful to determine whether there is an internal derangement, such as meniscus dislocation, or to evaluate for abnormal movement of the joint itself. Dental radiographs or CT can be used to examine odontogenic causes of pain. Symptoms of trigeminal neuralgia are evaluated using MRI to identify any abnormalities along the trigeminal nerve course. Structural abnormalities that may cause trigeminal neuralgia include mass effect on the cisternal segment of the trigeminal nerve secondary to a vascular loop or cerebellopontine angle mass and abnormalities within the brainstem affecting the trigeminal nerve nucleus such as multiple sclerosis, infection, or tumor. Acute optic neuritis and orbital pseudotumor are among the secondary causes of orbital headache and facial pain, and are both evaluated using MRI with contrast to study the orbits and optic nerve pathways. Enhancement, edema, and swelling may be seen in the optic nerve during acute optic neuritis. Orbital pseudotumor is an idiopathic orbital inflammatory disorder that may be limited to the orbit or may demonstrate intracranial extension to involve the cavernous sinus, which is then designated Tolosa-Hunt syndrome. Imaging findings of inflammation, enhancement, and occasionally a mass can be seen involving different structures within the orbit.

SUMMARY

When deciding to perform imaging for headache, it is important to consider many factors including the pretest probability, prevalence of diseases, sensitivity of imaging, and implications for treatment. For the first presentation of a headache or a change in headache pattern, if the characteristics do not perfectly fit a primary headache type, imaging may be indicated according to the ICHD-2 criteria to exclude a secondary cause before a primary headache is diagnosed. The value of negative imaging should not be underestimated in the cost-benefit analysis, which often only takes into account number needed to treat or likelihood of finding a significant treatable abnormality. One study has shown that some groups of patients are less likely to overuse other parts of the health care system after negative neuroimaging.[59] Further studies with stronger methodologies, finer differentiation of acute and chronic headache presentations, more advanced imaging technology, among other factors, can improve decision making on when to use imaging and assess the impact of imaging on patient satisfaction and quality of life. In addition, functional MRI, MRS, and voxel-based morphometry MRI are only some of the neuroimaging techniques currently used in research to further understand the pathophysiology and mechanisms of headache.

In conclusion, although most headaches are a primary headache disorder with a benign course, imaging is an important part of the diagnostic evaluation to exclude the presence of a secondary cause of headache that could cause fatal results or severe neurologic morbidity. In headache patients without focal neurologic examination abnormalities, the yield of neuroimaging for significant intracranial findings is generally low. However, specific subgroups of headache patients and headache presentations can have much higher rates of significant intracranial abnormalities.

REFERENCES

1. Medina LS, D'Souza B, Vasconcellos E. Adults and children with headache: evidence-based diagnostic evaluation. Neuroimaging Clin N Am 2003;13(2): 225–35.
2. Evans RW. Diagnostic testing for the evaluation of headaches. Neurol Clin 1996; 14:1–26.
3. Jordan JE, Expert panel on neurologic imaging. Headache. AJNR Am J Neuroradiol 2007;28(9):1824–6.

4. Evans RW. Diagnostic testing for migraines and other primary headaches. Neurol Clin 2009;27:393–415.

5. Frishberg BM, Rosenberg JH, Matchar DB, et al. Evidence-based guidelines in the primary care setting: neuroimaging in patients with nonacute headache. Available at: http://www.aan.com/professionals/practice/pdfs/gl0088.pdr. Accessed October 30, 2012.

6. Demaerel P, Boelaert I, Wilms G, et al. The role of cranial computed tomography in the diagnostic work-up of headache. Headache 1996;36:347–8.

7. Dumas MD, Pexman W, Kreeft JH. Computed tomography evaluation of patients with chronic headache. Can Med Assoc J 1994;151:1447–52.

8. Sotaniemi KA, Rantala M, Pyhtinen J, et al. Clinical and CT correlates in the diagnosis of intracranial tumours. J Neurol Neurosurg Psychiatry 1991;54:645–7.

9. Wang HZ, Simonson TM, Greco WR, et al. Brain MR imaging in the evaluation of chronic headache in patients without other neurologic symptoms. Acad Radiol 2001;8(5):405–8.

10. Detsky ME, McDonald DR, Baerlocher MO, et al. Does this patient with headache have a migraine or need neuroimaging? JAMA 2006;296:1274–83.

11. Sempere AP, Porta-Etessam J, Medrano V, et al. Neuroimaging in the evaluation of patients with non-acute headache. Cephalalgia 2005;25(1):30–5.

12. Headache Classification Committee of the International Headache Society. The international classification of headache disorders. Cephalalgia 2004;24:1–160. Available at: http://ihs-classification.org/en/. Accessed October 30, 2012.

13. Silberstein SD. Practice parameter: evidence-based guidelines for migraine headache (an evidence-based review): report of the Quality Standards Subcommittee of the American Academy of Neurology. Neurology 2000;55(6):754–62.

14. Edlow JA, Panagos PD, Godwin SA, et al, American College of Emergency Physicians. Clinical policy: critical issues in the evaluation and management of adult patients presenting to the emergency department with acute headache. Ann Emerg Med 2008;52(4):407–36.

15. Jordan JE, Wippold FJ II, Cornelius RS, et al. Expert panel on neurologic imaging. ACR appropriateness criteria headache. Reston (VA): American College of Radiology (ACR); 2009. Available at: http://www.acr.org/Quality-Safety/Appropriateness-Criteria/Diagnostic/Neurologic-Imaging. Accessed October 30, 2012.

16. Sudlow C. US guidelines on neuroimaging in patients with non-acute headache: a commentary. J Neurol Neurosurg Psychiatry 2002;72(Suppl 2):ii16–8.

17. De Luca GC, Bartleson JD. When and how to investigate the patient with headache. Semin Neurol 2010;30(2):131–44.

18. Schaefer PW, Miller JC, Singhal AB, et al. Headache: when is neurologic imaging indicated? J Am Coll Radiol 2007;4(8):566–9.

19. Evans RW, Rozen TD, Mechtler L. Neuroimaging and other diagnostic testing in headache. In: Silberstein SD, Lipton RB, Dodick DW, editors. Wolff's headache and other head pain. 8th edition. New York: Oxford University Press; 2008. p. 63–93.

20. Evans RW. Migraine: a question and answer review. Med Clin North Am 2009; 93(2):245–62, vii.

21. Edlow JA. What are the unintended consequences of changing the diagnostic paradigm for subarachnoid hemorrhage after brain computed tomography to computed tomographic angiography in place of lumbar puncture? Acad Emerg Med 2010;17(9):991–5 [discussion: 996–7].

22. Samarasekera N, Smith C, Al-Shahi Salman R. The association between cerebral amyloid angiopathy and intracerebral haemorrhage: systematic review and meta-analysis. J Neurol Neurosurg Psychiatry 2012;83(3):275–81.

23. Knudsen KA, Rosand J, Karluk D, et al. Clinical diagnosis of cerebral amyloid angiopathy: validation of the Boston criteria. Neurology 2001;56(4):537–9.

24. Hart RG, Boop BS, Anderson DC. Oral anticoagulants and intracranial hemorrhage facts and hypotheses. Stroke 1995;26:1471–7.

25. Hart RG, Diener H, Yang S, et al. Intracranial hemorrhage in atrial fibrillation patients during anticoagulation with warfarin or dabigatran: the RE-LY Trial. Stroke 2012;43:1511–7.

26. Witmer CM, Raffini LJ, Manno CS. Utility of computed tomography of the head following head trauma in boys with haemophilia. Haemophilia 2007;13(5):560–6.

27. Chern JJ, Tsung AJ, Humphries W, et al. Clinical outcome of leukemia patients with intracranial hemorrhage. J Neurosurg 2011;115(2):268–72.

28. US Cancer Statistics Working Group. United States cancer statistics: 2006–2010 incidence and mortality Web-based report. Available at: http://www.cdc.gov/cancer/npcr/uscs. Accessed October 30, 2012.

29. Kernick DP, Ahmed F, Bahra A, et al. Imaging patients with suspected brain tumour: guidance for primary care. Br J Gen Pract 2008;58(557):880–5.

30. Edwards RJ, Britz GW, Marsh H. Chronic headaches due to occult hydrocephalus. J R Soc Med 2003;96(2):77–8.

31. Verdelho A, Ferro JM, Melo T, et al. Headache in acute stroke. A prospective study in the first 8 days. Cephalalgia 2008;28(4):346–54.

32. Vestergaard K, Andersen G, Nielsen MI, et al. Headache in stroke. Stroke 1993; 24(11):1621–4.

33. Diener HC, Katsarava Z, Weimar C. Headache associated with ischemic cerebrovascular disease. Rev Neurol (Paris) 2008;164(10):819–24.

34. Tentschert S, Wimmer R, Greisenegger S, et al. Headache at stroke onset in 2196 patients with ischemic stroke or transient ischemic attack. Stroke 2005;36(2): e1–3.

35. Laurell K, Lundström E. Migrainous infarction: aspects on risk factors and therapy. Curr Pain Headache Rep 2012;16(3):255–60.

36. Wolf ME, Szabo K, Griebe M, et al. Clinical and MRI characteristics of acute migrainous infarction. Neurology 2011;76(22):1911–7.

37. Rodallec MH, Marteau V, Gerber S, et al. Craniocervical arterial dissection: spectrum of imaging findings and differential diagnosis. Radiographics 2008;28(6): 1711–28.

38. Smetana GW, Shmerling RH. Does this patient have temporal arteritis? JAMA 2002;287(1):92–101.

39. Chew SS, Kerr NM, Danesh-Meyer HV. Giant cell arteritis. J Clin Neurosci 2009; 16(10):1263–8.

40. Fitzgerald AJ, Ironside JW, Summers DM, et al. Two cases of recurrent stroke in treated giant cell arteritis: diagnostic and therapeutic dilemmas. J Clin Rheumatol 2010;16(5):225–8.

41. Ducros A, Boukobza M, Porcher R, et al. The clinical and radiological spectrum of reversible cerebral vasoconstriction syndrome. A prospective series of 67 patients. Brain 2007;130(Pt 12):3091–101.

42. Ducros A. Reversible cerebral vasoconstriction syndrome. Lancet Neurol 2012; 11(10):906–17.

43. Zach V, Bezov D, Lipton RB, et al. Headache associated with moyamoya disease: a case story and literature review. J Headache Pain 2010;11(1):79–82.

44. Ramchandren S, Cross BJ, Liebeskind DS. Emergent headaches during pregnancy: correlation between neurologic examination and neuroimaging. AJNR Am J Neuroradiol 2007;28(6):1085–7.

45. Delfyett WT, Fetzer DT. Imaging of neurologic conditions during pregnancy and the perinatal period. Neurol Clin 2012;30:791–822.
46. Lewis DW, Ashwal S, Dahl G, et al. Practice parameter: evaluation of children and adolescents with recurrent headaches: report of the Quality Standards Subcommittee of the American Academy of Neurology and the Practice Committee of the Child Neurology Society. Neurology 2002;59(4):490–8.
47. Lee VW, Antonacci V, Tilak S, et al. Intracranial mass lesions: sequential thallium and gallium scintigraphy in patients with AIDS. Radiology 1999;211(2):507–12.
48. Schievink WI. Spontaneous spinal cerebrospinal fluid leaks and intracranial hypotension. JAMA 2006;295(19):2286–96.
49. Wendl CM, Schambach F, Zimmer C, et al. CT myelography for the planning and guidance of targeted epidural blood patches in patients with persistent spinal CSF leakage. AJNR Am J Neuroradiol 2012;33(3):541–4.
50. Akbar JJ, Luetmer PH, Schwartz KM, et al. The role of MR myelography with intrathecal gadolinium in localization of spinal CSF leaks in patients with spontaneous intracranial hypotension. AJNR Am J Neuroradiol 2012;33(3):535–40.
51. Luetmer PH, Schwartz KM, Eckel LJ, et al. When should I do dynamic CT myelography? Predicting fast spinal CSF leaks in patients with spontaneous intracranial hypotension. AJNR Am J Neuroradiol 2012;33(4):690–4.
52. Hoxworth JM, Trentman TL, Kotsenas AL, et al. The role of digital subtraction myelography in the diagnosis and localization of spontaneous spinal CSF leaks. AJR Am J Roentgenol 2012;199(3):649–53.
53. Reynolds MR, Willie JT, Zipfel GJ, et al. Sexual intercourse and cerebral aneurysmal rupture: potential mechanisms and precipitants. J Neurosurg 2011; 114(4):969–77.
54. Yeh YC, Fuh JL, Chen SP, et al. Clinical features, imaging findings and outcomes of headache associated with sexual activity. Cephalalgia 2010;30(11):1329–35.
55. Wang SJ, Fuh JL. The "other" headaches: primary cough, exertion, sex, and primary stabbing headaches. Curr Pain Headache Rep 2010;14(1):41–6.
56. Frese A, Eikermann A, Frese K, et al. Headache associated with sexual activity: demography, clinical features, and comorbidity. Neurology 2003;61(6):796–800.
57. Davis PC, Brunberg JA, De La Paz RL, et al. Expert panel on neurologic imaging. ACR appropriateness criteria head trauma. Reston (VA): American College of Radiology (ACR); 2008. Available at: http://www.acr.org/Quality-Safety/Appropriateness-Criteria/Diagnostic/Neurologic-Imaging. Accessed October 30, 2012.
58. Jagoda AS, Bazarian JJ, Bruns JJ Jr, et al, American College of Emergency Physicians. Clinical policy: neuroimaging and decisionmaking in adult mild traumatic brain injury in the acute setting. Ann Emerg Med 2008;52(6):714–48.
59. Howard L, Wessely S, Leese M, et al. Are investigations anxiolytic or anxiogenic? A randomised controlled trial of neuroimaging to provide reassurance in chronic daily headache. J Neurol Neurosurg Psychiatry 2005;76(11):1558–64.

Managing and Treating Headache of Cervicogenic Origin

Maunak V. Rana, MD[a,b,*]

KEYWORDS

- Headache • Cervicogenic • Cephalgia • Occipital neuralgia • Migraine • Whiplash

KEY POINTS

- The term *cervicogenic headache* describes a clinical syndrome of chronic, typically unilateral headaches derived from the neck structures.
- Cervicogenic headaches may be seen in patients with other conditions, including myofascial pain, occipital neuralgia, and migraine headaches.
- The diagnosis of a cervicogenic headache is a predominantly clinical one because no laboratory or radiographic studies consistently confirm the syndrome.
- Techniques of treating a cervicogenic headache include pharmacotherapy, physical and manipulation therapy, interventional injections, and surgical procedures via a multidisciplinary approach.

INTRODUCTION

Cervicogenic headache (CGH) describes a syndrome of secondary hemi-cranial cephalgia thought to be originating from the structures in the cervical spine. Skeletal, connective tissues, and neurovascular structures may be the source of the discomfort in patients. Controversy exists as to the existence of this clinical diagnosis, with some describing the relationship between cervical structures and headache pain as "unproven and often dubious."[1]

Clinicians are faced with a true diagnostic dilemma because of the multitude of structures that may be the causative factor of this headache pain. Additionally, there is no definite test or radiographic finding that definitely leads to a diagnosis of CGH. Physicians from all scopes of practice, from generalists to specialists, will need to be familiar with this syndrome because its prevalence ranges widely throughout the population and may be seen across various disciplines. Some estimates highlight

Disclosures: None relevant to this article.
a Chicago Anesthesia Pain Specialists, Chicago, IL, USA; b Department of Anesthesiology, Advocate Illinois Masonic Medical Center, 836 West Wellington Avenue, #4815, Chicago, IL 60657, USA
* Department of Anesthesiology, Advocate Illinois Masonic Medical Center, University of Illinois-Chicago, 836 West Wellington Avenue, #4815, Chicago, IL 60657.
E-mail address: maunakr@gmail.com

Med Clin N Am 97 (2013) 267–280
http://dx.doi.org/10.1016/j.mcna.2012.11.003
0025-7125/13/$ – see front matter © 2013 Elsevier Inc. All rights reserved.

0.5% to 4.0%[2] of the population as suffering from CGH. In patients with headaches overall, an estimated 15% to 20% may have CGH.

The quality of life (QOL) of patients with CGH is significantly affected. A study used the Medical Outcomes Study Short Form Questionnaire (SF-36) to evaluate the QOL of patients with CGH, migraine, and tension-type headaches.[3] Patients with CGH were more affected regarding their perception of bodily pain and role limitations and physical functioning than were patients with other headache types. The investigators suggest that the chronicity of CGH may account for differences in QOL reported by patients.[3] A systematic approach to characterize and attempt diagnosis is, therefore, required. After excluding other sources of a headache that may be life threatening in nature, treatment can then be instituted.

HISTORY

Sjaastad and colleagues[4] first mentioned the term *cervicogenic headache* in the literature in 1983 to describe a subset of patients with headaches whose origin of pain develops in the cervical spine. Previously, it was thought that a description of headaches with a source from the neck region was described in 1853; however, the earliest description that is currently accessible is credited to Holmes from a published report in 1913. The investigator in that article noted that tender areas in the cervical muscles could lead to the development of headaches.[5]

Other descriptions noted occipital pain manifesting with auditory and visual alterations as part of "posterior cervical sympathetic syndrome."[5]

The term *occipital neuralgia* was devised after the work of Haddon, who described a suboccipital discomfort that was accentuated by palpation over the greater occipital nerve (GON) with radiation to the temporal region. Patients were noted to have nausea/vomiting, visual changes, and resolution of their symptoms with nerve blockade.[5]

In 1949, Hunter and Mayfield described a group of patients suffering from migraine-like symptoms who had benefit from their complaints after upper cervical nerve blockade. C2 nerve blockade was found to be completely effective in treating the patients in this series; GON block was less effective at providing relief of symptoms.[5]

The Swiss neurologist Barschi-Rochaix contributed to the linking of cervical structures to headache pain.[5] The identification of cephalgia status after cervical spine trauma along with aberration of the cervical facet joints was highlighted as causative factors for headache pain. The term *cervical migraine* was coined based on this work.

Josey, in 1949, described a series of 6 cases of mechanically precipitated cervical headaches, unilateral in location.[6] Maigne, in 1976, also noted the presence of cephalgia originating from the neck structures, describing a "cervical headache."[5]

Various investigators also historically observed the contribution of the cervical disk to headache.[5–7]

In 1983, in their evaluation of patients with headache, Sjaastad and colleagues[4] suggested the presence of a unique CGH in patients with cervical spine complaints. The International Headache Society (IHS) did not recognize this diagnosis in its 1988 classification system by not including a distinct CGH designation.

Sjaastad founded the Cervicogenic Headache International Study Group (CHIG) in 1987 to describe and elucidate criteria for the diagnosis of this condition. In 1994, the International Association for the Study of Pain (IASP) presented diagnostic criteria, formally recognizing CGH.[8]

Subsequent criteria have been revised, and the IHS in the International Classification of Headache Disorders[9] has noted CGH.

EPIDEMIOLOGY

Prevalence estimates range from 0.4% to 2.5% of the general population to 15% to 20% of patients with chronic headaches,[10] making this syndrome a significant issue. Others[11,12] have noted that this may be present in up to 34% of patients with headaches. CGH affects patients with a mean age of 42.9 years, has a 4:1 female disposition, and tends to be chronic in nature.[11,12]

PATIENT PRESENTATION

The discomfort from CGH may be of variable onset and duration,[11-13] making the diagnosis and treatment of this condition difficult.

Patients with CGH typically present with a unilateral headache located in the suboccipital/occipital region that travels to the temporal and periorbital regions[13] as depicted in **Fig. 1**. Bilateral presentation may also occur.[14] Discomfort may also be noted in the parietal and frontal portions of the head and the upper extremity. The headache is side locked and does not switch between the sides.[13] Additionally, the cervical spine range of motion is decreased; during cervical spine motion, the headache is precipitated. This aspect of patient presentation point regarding headache provocation can allow for the distinction between other headache types.[13] Patients may present with nausea/vomiting, photophobia, neck and arm pain, along with cephalgia.

DIAGNOSTIC CRITERIA

The IHS classification[9] is presented in **Box 1**. In analyzing this scheme, a few points are to be noted. The IHS places a caveat with criteria B noting that "Tumors, fractures, infections and rheumatoid arthritis of the upper cervical spine have not been validated formally as causes of headache, but are nevertheless accepted as valid causes when demonstrated to be so in individual cases."[9] Furthermore, the IHS criteria do not include cervical spondylosis as a cause of CGH, contradicting the historical work highlighted previously. Also, the criteria do not include myofascial trigger points in the definition of CGH, instead categorizing these patients as suffering from tension-type headaches, regardless of the source of the pain.

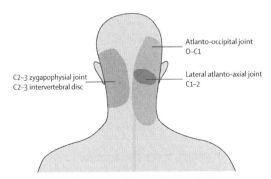

Fig. 1. Pattern of CGH pain. The location of discomfort in the head and neck region and the origin in the cervical spine of discomfort. (*Reprinted from* Bogduk N, Govind J. Cervicogenic headache: an assessment of the evidence on clinical diagnosis, invasive tests, and treatment. Lancet Neurol 2009;8:961; with permission.)

Box 1
IHS classification of CGH

1. Pain, referred from a source in the neck and perceived in one or more regions of the head and/or face, fulfilling criteria 3 and 4

2. Clinical, laboratory, and/or imaging evidence of a disorder or lesion within the cervical spine or soft tissues of the neck known to be or generally accepted as a valid cause of headaches

3. Evidence that the pain can be attributed to the neck disorder or lesion based on at least one of the following

   a. Demonstration of clinical signs that implicate a source of pain in the neck[2]

   b. Abolition of the headache following diagnostic blockade of a cervical structure or its nerve supply using placebo or other adequate controls

4. Pain resolves within 3 months after successful treatment of the causative disorder or lesion

---

The IHS requires pain relief of 90% or more reduction in pain to a level of less than 5 on a 100-point visual analog scale and mentions a time frame for resolution of pain. This final portion of the criteria would define CGH as an acute process rather than a chronic, reoccurring syndrome.

The CHIG classification system[4,13] (**Box 2**) presents more comprehensive criteria for inclusion in this diagnosis. It includes a graded description of signs, symptoms, and response to therapies. Specifically, this classification system highlights that CGH must be unilateral without side shift. It is less specific on etiologic factors that may cause the headache along with no mention of time duration in comparison with the IHS classification. The 2 systems provide complementary and synergistic information to clinicians treating patients with CGH.

ANATOMIC CONSIDERATIONS

According to proponents of the existence of CGH, symptoms may be caused by any potential structure in the cervical region: osseous, soft tissue ligaments, neural, and vascular structures.[14–19] Rather than isolated structures accounting for pain, concomitant aberration in any of the structures may also act in concert to lead to the discomfort. A discussion of cranial to caudal structures that may lead to the pain is important for practitioners to consider.

NEUROANATOMY

The trigeminocervical nucleus in the upper cervical spinal cord receives afferent impulses from cranial nerve V (trigeminal nerve) and the superior 3 cervical spinal nerves (**Fig. 2**).[14,16] The nucleus may serve as a relay station for input from distal areas leading to nociceptive sensation in the areas innervated by the trigeminal nerve yet originating in the cervical region, thereby culminating in headache symptoms. A suggestion based on feline neuroanatomy is made for this bidirectional cervicotrigeminal relay activating the trigeminovascular system, which could lead to a possible migraine portion of CGH.[12] An example of this referred discomfort occurs with noxious stimulation of the GON with resultant excitation of supratentorial afferents.

BONY PATHOLOGY

The atlanto-occipital joint (AO) serves as the segue between the cranium and the appendicular skeleton (**Fig. 3**).[14,15,18] This synovial-lined condylar joint allows for

---

Box 2
CHIG diagnostic criteria

Major Criteria

1. Symptoms and signs of neck involvement

    a. Precipitation of comparable symptoms by

        i. Neck movement and/or sustained, awkward head positioning, and/or

        ii. External pressure over the upper cervical or occipital region

            1. Restriction of range of motion in the neck

            2. Ipsilateral neck, shoulder, or arm pain

2. Confirmatory evidence by diagnostic anesthetic block

3. Unilaterality of the head pain, without side shift

Head Pain Characteristics

4. Moderate-severe, nonthrobbing pain, usually starting in the neck

    a. Episodes of varying duration or fluctuating, continuous pain

Other Characteristics of some Importance

5. Only marginal or lack of effect of indomethacin

6. Only marginal or lack of effect of ergotamine and sumatriptan

7. Female gender

8. Not infrequent history of head or indirect neck trauma, usually of more than medium severity

Other Features of Lesser Importance

9. Various attack-related phenomena, only occasionally present, and/or moderately expressed when present:

    a. Nausea

    b. Phonophobia and photophobia

    c. Dizziness

    d. Ipsilateral blurred vision

    e. Difficulties swallowing

    f. Ipsilateral edema, mostly in the periocular area

---

flexion and extension as well as slight lateral rotation of the cranium on the cervical spine. The dorsal ramus of the C1 nerve, the suboccipital nerve, is responsible for innervating the AO joint. Pathology of this region may lead to discomfort noted in the suboccipital region along with migrainelike symptoms.[14,15,18]

The atlanto-axial (AA) joint (see **Fig. 3**) is a complex of 2 lateral and a median articulations. The lateral portion of the joint allows for a gliding motion and the median provides a pivot of the dens and the arch of the atlas.[14,15,18] The joint complex is innervated by the C2 dorsal root ganglion (DRG). This neural structure is particularly vulnerable to injury because of a ligamentous covering (atlantoepistropic ligament) as opposed to a bony covering.[14,16,17]

C2 neuralgia may lead to radiating holocranial discomfort. Ocular symptoms, including lacrimation or conjunctival injection, may occur. Additionally, vascular irritation of the C2 ganglion may lead to headache symptoms.[17]

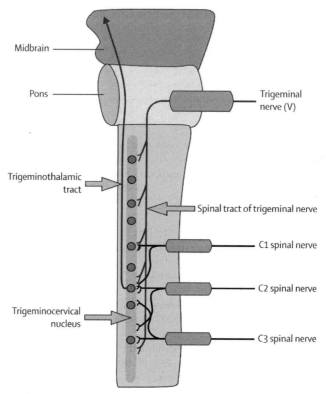

Fig. 2. Pathway of referred pain from cervical spine to head. The trigeminocervical nucleus in the upper portion of the spinal cord serves as a relay station for afferent fibers from the trigeminal nerve and the first 3 cervical spinal nerves. The bidirectional signal pathway accounts for the sensation of pain from the cervical spine to cranial areas receiving input from the trigeminal nerve. (*Reprinted from* Bogduk N, Govind J. Cervicogenic headache: an assessment of the evidence on clinical diagnosis, invasive tests, and treatment. Lancet Neurol 2009;8:959–68; with permission.)

This joint can be a source of discomfort in patients with CGH. It has been reported that 16% of patients with occipital headaches have the lateral AA joint as the source.[14,19] Reports exist in the literature of reproduction of pain in the occipital region with filling of the joint.[20,21]

Headache symptoms may be treated with a nerve block, thus alleviating pain allowing for diagnostic and therapeutic benefit.[18]

Some have opined that the C2-C3 joint is the critical spinal level for the generation of CGH (see **Fig. 3**).[19,20] Occipital and upper cervical discomfort has been elicited by injecting the C2-3 joint. A branch of the C2DRG also supplies[21,22] this level. The dynatomes, areas of sensitivity caused by aberrant nerve root function, do not overlap in this region and are distinct from dermatomal mapping.[21] The C2 dynatome has been noted to range from the occipital region to the vertex of the cranium. The C3 dynatome has a more craniofacial and upper cervical coverage area. Pathologic abnormalities in these regions can lead to CGH. As a result, patients may describe a deep, dull, aching discomfort in the occipital or upper cervical region.

Reports in the literature exist of a favorable response to intra-articular joint injections as both diagnostic and therapeutic options.[22]

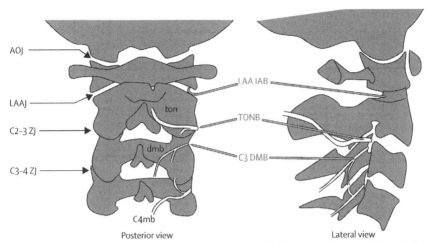

Posterior view   Lateral view

Fig. 3. Posterior/lateral view of the joints and nerves of the cervical spine. AOJ, AO joint, also known as C0-C1 joint level; C2-3ZJ, C2-C3 zygapophyseal joint; C3-C4 ZJ, C3-C4 zygapophyseal joint; C3DMB, C3 dorsal ramus medial branch block location; C4mb, C4 dorsal ramus medial branch; DMB, deep medial branch; LAA IAB, lateral atlanto-axial joint intra-articular block; LAAJ, lateral atlanto-axial joint, also known as C1-C2 joint level; ton, third occipital nerve; TONB, third occipital nerve block location. (*Reprinted from* Bogduk N, Govind J. Cervicogenic headache: an assessment of the evidence on clinical diagnosis, invasive tests, and treatment. Lancet Neurol 2009;8:959–68; with permission.)

CERVICAL DISK DISEASE

Cervical disk disease has been implicated in the generation of CGH.[23] A possible mechanism of discogenic pain was advocated by Bogduk and colleagues[24] concerning the sinuvertebral nerves. In a series of 173 patients undergoing provocative discography over a 12-year period in the cervical spine, the C2/3 level pain provocation was in the occiput and cranium as opposed to other levels evaluated.[23]

Cervical disk pathology may be seen in patients presenting with CGH, but the clinical utility of the finding is of uncertain value. A case report[25] describes a patient with chronic CGH who underwent lower cervical disk surgery with subsequent resolution of headache symptoms. Another study[26] mentions the role of lower cervical spine pathology and CGH. Twelve patients with IHS criteria for CGH underwent cervical spine surgery for disk prolapse. Eighty percent of these patients had improvement or resolution of their discomfort. The supposed mechanism suggested by the investigators is an anatomic connection between the lower cervical nerve roots and the cervical trigeminal nucleus.[26]

DIFFERENTIAL DIAGNOSIS

A complete history and physical examination, including directed musculoskeletal and thorough neurologic, is required in the evaluation of patients. Palpation of the cervical spine may reveal discomfort in patients. Occipital tenderness may be elicited with palpation over the areas of the greater/lesser occipital nerves. Palpation over the C2-C4 facet joint levels may also elicit pain in patients.

Because the number of structures that can lead to CGH symptoms is great, it is crucial for the practicing clinician to discount other causes that would warrant further urgent treatment.

Arnold-Chiari type I is an inferior herniation of the cerebellar tonsils through the foramen magnum, potentially leading to hydrocephalus and mimicking CGH.[27]

Posterior fossa tumors may also present similar to CGH. The physical location of the tumor is proximate to the occipital region. Additionally, the dura mater receives innervation by the branches of the superior cervical nerves.[17,19]

Vascular aneurysms particularly deleterious if undiagnosed can also mimic CGH. If suspected, magnetic resonance angiography may be required for diagnostic purposes. Upper cervical neuropathy caused by inflammatory or medical conditions (malignancy, lupus, rheumatoid arthritis, endocrine disease) may also mimic CGH because of aberrant nerve function.[16,19]

Whiplash Injury

Sudden cervical acceleration-deceleration injury of the cervical spine leading to hyperextension may result in an entity known as whiplash syndrome. This entity may be seen after cervical spine trauma, most commonly after motor vehicle collisions. A graded classification system exists for triage of patients presented by the Quebec Task Force based on symptoms and degree of neuraxial injury.[28]

Between 50% and 75% of patients diagnosed with whiplash injury may have CGH. The C2-C3 level is the putative level involved in headache symptoms secondary to whiplash injury (cervical acceleration/deceleration injury) sustained during motor vehicle collisions, present in 27% of patients according to one published study.[29] Others point out that few patients with cervical whiplash develop chronic headaches.[30–32] Treatment may involve nonsteroidal analgesics, muscle relaxants, and physical therapy.[29]

Migraine

Migraine headaches may be confused with CGH because of similar features.[30,33] Migraine traits may be noted in some patients with CGH. CGH may also possibly occur in any or all of the 3 phases of a migraine attack: prodrome, active headache, and recovery. In one study, 64% of patients with migraines had neck discomfort during an attack.[34] Another study of patients with migraines noted that 98% of patients with a unilateral headache during the migraine attack had ipsilateral cervical spine pain.[35,36]

Factors differentiating the two have been proposed.[30] The results of the evaluations of patients have shown that CGH is more likely to be side locked unilaterally regarding symptoms, more likely to cause radiation of symptoms to the ipsilateral extremity, and be provoked by palpation or changes in posture. Migraines have a greater female preponderance; may be side shifting; and are more likely to lead to nausea, vomiting, photophobia, and phonophobia.[30,33]

Occipital Neuralgia

Occipital neuralgia (ON) describes headaches in the areas surrounded by the greater or lesser occipital nerves. The GON is a branch of the dorsal ramus of C2, and the lesser occipital nerve (LON) is a branch of the dorsal portion of C3.[8]

The C2-C3 level is the putative level involved in headache symptoms secondary to whiplash injury. This cervical level is innervated by the superficial branch of the dorsal ramus of C3, the third occipital nerve (TON).[14] This nerve is a particularly tenacious nerve that requires the placement of 3 needles to block the nerve: superior to the joint, at the level of the joint, and inferior to the level of the C2-C3 joint.

After successful nerve block, patients may undergo radiofrequency ablation (RF) for potentially longer-term relief of symptoms. In one series, 88% of patients had TON CGH relief with RF.[37]

CGH has been treated with RF at facet joints as well as the cervical disks.[14]

Surgical intervention may also be required for the treatment of ON. This intervention may take the form of an occipital nerve stimulator,[38,39] which is a percutaneously placed electrode connected to a generator for neuromodulation of the painful region. Results from published studies show between 75% and 88% of patients have more than a 50% reduction in severity and frequency of headache pain.[38,39]

Additionally, neurosurgical nerve root decompression of affected levels may be an option. In refractory cases of intractable ON, C2 ganglionectomy was performed.[40] Sixty-six percent of patients had good to excellent relief on a mean follow-up of 5.6 years. The average pain score reduction with this therapy was 5 on a visual analog scale.

The investigators of this study pointed out that in a pathway of treating patients with this debilitating condition, occipital nerve stimulation should occur *before* ganglionectomy because the former is more of a neuromodulatory technique as opposed to the latter lesioning procedure.

Myofascial Pain

Soft tissue and muscular aberration in the cervical region may also present as CGH.[41] Alterations in muscle tone and strength in patients with CGH manifesting as an "Upper Crossed Syndrome"[42]: weak rhomboid/lower trapezius and cervical flexors; tight suboccipitalis, upper trapezius, and pectorals may be present. Myofascial pain caused by trigger points in the suboccipital, prevertebral, and cervical muscles may result. Typically, the sternocleidomastoid, trapezius, semispinalis, splenius, and semispinalis muscles may be involved.[42]

DIAGNOSTIC STUDIES

Imaging of the brain and cervical spine does not reliably provide information for confirming the diagnosis of CGH.[16] Opinion varies on the efficacy of radiographic findings in patients with CGH. One study evaluating patients with CGH showed no difference in functional (flexion/extension views) of the cervical spine, but computer-based measurements showed statistically significant hypomobility of the AO joint and hypermobility of the C6/7 segment.[43] Magnetic resonance imaging (MRI) studies do not typically show consistent variation between patients with CGH and control patients.[44]

In a study of 42 patients (22 with CGH according to the CIGH criteria and 20 similar control patients), 45% of patients with CGH had evidence of disk bulging in the cervical spine, with 45% of control patients also having disk bulge. The distribution of disk bulging across the cervical spine also did not differ between the two groups. MRI may not have a significant role in diagnosing CGH but may be of benefit in excluding conditions that may be life threatening. Biologic markers have also been evaluated highlighting the calcitonin gene-related peptide (CGRP); this has been inconclusive.[45]

Bovim[46] studied the pressure pain threshold (PPT) measurement as a model for evaluating pain sensitivity in patients with headaches. Patients with CGH were compared with migraines, tension headaches, and normal controls. The patients with CGH had a statistically significant lower PPT as measured by a pressure algometer. The investigator of the study suggests that this difference in threshold sensitivity may add credence to the belief of the distinct nature of CGH compared with other headaches.

Diagnostic interventional injections have provided benefit in diagnosis and treatment of the pain of CGH as mentioned previously.[14,18,47–49]

MEDICAL MANAGEMENT

There are no current medications approved by the Food and Drug Administration (FDA) for use in patients with CGH. Patients have been tried on a multi-modal regimen including antidepressants, antiepileptic medications, nonsteroidal antiinflammatory drugs (NSAIDS), migraine-abortive agents, muscle relaxants, and GABAergic agents, with varying degrees of relief.[16] The practicing clinician should be aware of the risks and benefits of various therapies. Patients may require agents individually or in combination for relief of their symptoms.

INTERVENTIONAL TREATMENT

Naja and colleagues[47] have described the benefit of occipital nerve block for CGH and noted the improvement of symptoms. The occipital nerve block, however, was performed with palpation over the location of the GON, which results in a field block rather than a specific, precise intervention.

Anthony[12] presented findings on the benefit of depot methylprednisolone deposited in the region of the GON and LON in treating CGH. Ninety-four percent of patients with CGH achieved relief of headache symptoms for a mean of 23.5 days.

Bovim[48] presented data on the efficacy of cervical nerve injections and cervical facet injections. GON was noted to be effective. The C2 nerve was noted to be most efficacious in decreasing CGH followed by the injection of the C2/3 facet level. The investigators note that cervical nerve injections distal to C3 would probably offer no clinical benefit.

Another study evaluated the deep cervical plexus block (C2-C4) for the treatment of CGH and found that this injection was effective in decreasing pain for 3 months.[49]

RF has been used for CGH with varying degrees of success. Stovner and colleagues[50] noted that RF for CGH has a maximum benefit of 3 months of relief and likely should not be recommended. Another report suggests RF is a viable option.[51]

Pulsed RF (PRF) has been described in the treatment of CGH because this is a neuromodulatory rather than a neuroablative technique. A case series presented 2 patients who underwent PRF of C2 DRG for the treatment of CGH with 100% relief for 6 months.[52] In one study, 50% of patients had relief for at least 2 months; 44% of patients had relief at 1 year after lateral atlantoaxial joint radiofrequency.[52,53]

Cervical epidural steroid injections have also been evaluated for patients with CGH.[54] A European study showed a benefit with short-term (12 hours) and medium-term (4 weeks) relief with less benefit over the long term. Patients in this study did not receive an MRI of the cervical spine before epidural injection. Also, epidurals were performed without the use of fluoroscopic guidance to ascertain accurate epidural spread.[55]

Additionally, only 40 mg was administered during the procedure at the lower cervical levels. Assuming that the pathologic level for CGH is at the C2-3 level, the extent of the spread of the corticosteroid to the level of interest it is unclear without fluoroscopic guidance.

BOTOX INJECTION

Botox is a purified extract of onabotulinum toxin A that has been used for cosmetic and analgesic purposes. It has recently received FDA approval for use in patients with migraine headaches. Case reports showed a benefit of Botox A injections in the occipital, cranial, and cervical regions in patients with CGH and migraine symptoms.[56]

A review of the literature[57] did not show any benefit in randomized controlled trials of the evaluation of Botox in headaches, with some benefit noted in individual case reports.

For CGH, 2 randomized controlled trials (one positive study and one negative study) were included. Two studies addressing chronic neck pain were included in this review. Both studies did not reveal significant effects.[57–59]

NONINTERVENTIONAL/NONPHARMACOLOGIC APPROACHES

Physiotherapy is a viable treatment option for patients with CGH to enhance recovery and decrease the likelihood of the return of symptoms.[16,59–63] Therapy includes joint mobilization, range of motion, cervical traction, soft tissue massage, myofascial release, muscle strengthening, and posture/body mechanics adjustments.

Soft tissue manipulation and spinal manipulative therapy (SMT) is an option to adjust flexibility and to decrease muscle tightness.[60,61] One study noted that SMT was 50% more likely to improved pain scores in patients with CGH than light massage.[62]

SUMMARY

CGH is a common entity that has been assessed historically in various medical disciplines. Currently, CGH is a controversial topic whose existence has supporters and naysayers. The difficulty evaluating CGH is caused by a lack of objective findings on imaging and biologic tests. Patients present with pain but often with a lack of hard, concrete physical findings.

Other clinical diagnoses may confound the clinical presentation of patients. The concomitant presence of ON and migraine headaches has been noted in the literature. Positive analgesia after interventional techniques remains the major way to consider the diagnosis in potential patients with headaches.

Although the IHS has acknowledged CGH as a secondary headache in its diagnostic schema, more research, specifically randomized double-blinded evaluations of patients with CGH, are required. These data would be deemed as objective gold-standard evidence to lead us from controversy to collaborative agreement regarding the fate of CGH. What is certain regarding CGH is that a cooperative effort should be considered in the treatment of the patients between evaluating physicians, interventional pain physicians, surgeons, and physical therapy providers. This multidisciplinary effort can lead to the effective management of CGH.

REFERENCES

1. Edmeads J. The cervical spine and headache. Neurology 1988;38:1874–8.
2. Sjaastad O, Bakketeig LS. Prevalence of cervicogenic headache: Vaga study of headache epidemiology. Acta Neurol Scand 2008;117:170–83.
3. van Suijiekom HA, Lame I, Stomp-van den Berg SG, et al. Quality of life of patients with cervicogenic headache: a comparison with control subjects and patients with migraine or tension-type headache. Headache 2003;43:1034–41.
4. Sjaastad O, Saunte C, Hovdahl H, et al. "Cervicogenic" headache. An hypothesis. Cephalalgia 1983;3:249.
5. Antonaci F, Bono G, Mauri M, et al. Concepts leading to the definition of the term cervicogenic headache: a historical overview. J Headache Pain 2005;6(6):462–6.
6. Vincent M, Luna RA. Cervicogenic headache. Josey's cases revisited. Arq Neuro-psiquiatr 1997;55(4):841–8.

7. Jull G. Diagnosis of cervicogenic headache. J Man Manip Ther 2006;14(3): 136–8.

8. Merskey H, Bogduk N, editors. Classification of chronic pain. Descriptions of chronic pain syndromes and definitions of pain terms. Cervicogenic headache. 2nd edition. Seattle (WA): IASP; 1994.

9. IHS headache classification. Available at: http://ihs-classification.org/en/02_klassifikation/03_teil2/11.02.01_cranial.html. Accessed November, 2012.

10. Haldeman S, Dagenais S. Cervicogenic headaches: a critical review. Spine 2001; 1(1):31–46.

11. Nilsson N. The prevalence of cervicogenic headache in a random sample of 20-59 year olds. Spine 1995;20:1884–8.

12. Anthony M. Cervicogenic headache: prevalence and response to local steroid therapy. Clin Exp Rheumatol 2000;18(Suppl 19):59–64.

13. Sjaastad O, Fredriksen TA, Pfaffenrath V. Cervicogenic headache: diagnostic criteria. The Cervicogenic Headache International Study Group. Headache 1998;38(6):442–5.

14. Narouze S. Cervicogenic headache. In: Benzon HT, Raja SN, Liu SS, et al, editors. Essentials of pain medicine. 3rd edition. Philadelphia: Elsevier; 2011. p. 278–82.

15. Dreyfuss P, Michaelsen M, Fletcher D. Atlanto-occipital and lateral atlanto-axial joint pain patterns. Spine 1994;19:125–32.

16. Biondi DM. Cervicogenic headache: a review of diagnostic and treatment strategies. J Am Osteopath Assoc 2005;105(4 Suppl 2):S18–22.

17. Jansen J, Bardosi A, Hildebrandt J, et al. Cervicogenic, hemicranial attacks associated with vascular irritation or compression of the cervical nerve root C2. Pain 1989;39:203–12.

18. Racz GB, Anderson SR, Sizer PS, et al. Atlantaoccipital and atlantoaxial injections in the treatment of headache and neck pain. In: Waldman SD, editor. Interventional pain management. 2nd edition. Philadelphia: WB Saunders; 2001. p. 295–307.

19. Bogduk N. Cervicogenic headache: anatomical basis and pathophysiological mechanisms. Curr Pain Headache Rep 2001;5:382–6.

20. Meloche J, Bergeron Y, Bellavance A, et al. Painful intervertebral dysfunction: Robert Maigne's original contribution to headache of cervical origin. The Quebec Headache Study Group. Headache 1993;33:328–34.

21. Dwyer A, Aprill C, Bogduk N. Cervical zygapophyseal joint pain patterns I: a study of normal volunteers. Spine 1990;15:447–53.

22. Narouze SN, Casanova J, Mekhail N. The longitudinal effectiveness of lateral atlanto-axial intra-articular steroid injection in the management of cervicogenic headache. Pain Med 2007;8:184–8.

23. Grubb SA, Kelly CK. Cervical discography: clinical implications from 12 years of experience. Spine 2000;25:1382–9.

24. Bogduk N, Windsor M, Inglis A. The innervation of the cervical intervertebral discs. Spine 1988;13(1):2–8.

25. Michler RP, Bovim G, Sjaastad O. Disorders in the lower cervical spine. A cause of unilateral headache? A case report. Headache 1991;31:550–1.

26. Diener HC, Kaminski M, Stappert G, et al. Lower cervical disc prolapse may cause cervicogenic headache: a prospective study in patients undergoing surgery. Cephalalgia 2007;27:1050–4.

27. Stovner LJ. Headache associated with Chiari type I malformation. Headache 1993;33(4):175–81.

28. Freeman MD, Croft AC, Rossignol AM. "Whiplash associated disorders: redefining whiplash and its management" by the Quebec Task Force. A critical evaluation. Spine 1998;23(9):1043–9.
29. Yadla S, Gehret J, Campbell P, et al. A pain in the neck: review of cervicogenic headache and associated disorders. JHN Journal 2010;5(1):16–8.
30. Vincent M. Cervicogenic headache: a review comparison with migraine, tension-type headache, and whiplash. Curr Pain Headache Rep 2010;14:238–43.
31. Sjaastad O, Fredriksen TA, Baakesteig LS. Headache subsequent to whiplash. Curr Pain Headache Rep 2009;13:52–8.
32. Chou LH, Lenrow DA. Cervicogenic headache. Pain Physician 2002;5(2):215–25.
33. Sjaastad O, Bakketeig LS. Migraine without aura: comparison with cervicogenic headache. Vaga study of headache epidemiology. Acta Neurol Scand 2008;117:377–83.
34. Blau JN, MacGregor EA. Migraine and the neck. Headache 1994;34:88–90.
35. Kaniecki RG. Migraine and tension-type headache: an assessment of challenges in diagnosis. Neurology 2002;58(9 Suppl 16):S15–20.
36. Evers S. Comparison of cervicogenic headache with migraine. Cephalalgia 2008;28(Suppl 1):16–7.
37. Govind J, King W, Baily B, et al. Radiofrequency neurotomy for the treatment of third occipital headache. J Neurol Neurosurg Psychiatry 2003;74:88–93.
38. Aló KM, Holsheimer J. New trends in neuromodulation for the management of neuropathic pain. Neurosurgery 2002;50:690–704.
39. Popeney CA, Aló KM. Peripheral neurostimulation for the treatment of chronic, disabling transformed migraine. Headache 2003;43:369–75.
40. Pisapia JM, Bhowmick DA, Faber RE, et al. Salvage C2 ganglionectomy after C2 nerve root decompression provides similar pain relief as a single surgical procedure for intractable occipital neuralgia. World Neurosurg 2012;77(2):363–9.
41. Page P. Cervicogenic headaches: an evidence-led approach to clinical management. Int J Sports Phys Ther 2011;6(3):254–66.
42. Hall T, Briffa K, Hopper D. Clinical evaluation of cervicogenic headache: a clinical perspective. J Man Manip Ther 2008;16(2):73–80.
43. Pffafenrath V, Dandekar R, Mayer ET, et al. Cervicogenic headache: results of computer-based measurements of cervical spine mobility in 15 patients. Cephalalgia 1988;8(1):45–8.
44. Coskun O, Ucler S, Karakurum B, et al. Magnetic resonance imaging of patients with cervicogenic headache. Cephalalgia 2003;23(8):842–5.
45. Frese A, Evers S. Biological markers of cervicogenic headache. Cephalalgia 2008;28(Suppl 2):21–3.
46. Bovim G. Cervicogenic headache, migraine, and tension-type headache. Pressure-pain threshold measurements. Pain 1992;51:169–73.
47. Naja ZM, El-Rajab M, Al-Tannir MA, et al. Repetitive occipital nerve blockade for cervicogenic headache: expanded case report of 47 adults. Pain Pract 2006;6:278–84.
48. Bovim G, Berg R, Dale LG. Cervicogenic headache: anesthetic blockades of cervical nerves (C2-C5) and facet joint (C2/C3). Pain 1992;49:315–20.
49. Goldberg ME, Schwartzman RJ, Domsky R, et al. Deep cervical plexus block for the treatment of cervicogenic headache. Pain Physician 2008;11(6):849–54.
50. Stovner LJ, Kolstad F, Heide G. Radiofrequency denervation of facet joints C2-C6 in cervicogenic headache: a randomized double-blind, sham-controlled study. Cephalalgia 2004;24(10):821–30.

51. Lee JB, Park JY, Park J, et al. Clinical efficacy of radiofrequency cervical zygapophyseal neurotomy in patients with chronic cervicogenic headache. J Korean Med Sci 2007;22:326–9.
52. Zhang J, Shi DS, Wang R. Pulsed radiofrequency of the second cervical ganglion (C2) for the treatment of cervicogenic headache. J Headache Pain 2011;12(5): 569–71.
53. Halim W, Chua NH, Vissers KC. Long-term pain relief in patients with cervicogenic headaches after pulsed radiofrequency application into the lateral atlantoaxial (C1-2) joint using an anterolateral approach. Pain Pract 2010;10(4):267–71.
54. Martelletti P, DiSabato F, Granata M, et al. Epidural corticosteroid blockade in cervicogenic headache. Eur Rev Med Pharmacol Sci 1998;2:31–6.
55. Kurain J, Raghavan V, Raobaikady R. Minimizing the risk of dural puncture during cervical epidural steroid injection. Anesth Analg 2002;94(5):1366.
56. Hobson DE, Gladish DF. Botulinum toxin injection for cervicogenic headache. Headache 1997;37(4):253–5.
57. Oliver M, MacDonald J, Rajwani M. The use of botulinum neurotoxin type A (Botox) for headaches: a case review. J Can Chiropr Assoc 2006;50(4):263–70.
58. Sycha T, Kranz G, Auff E, et al. Botulinum toxin in the treatment of rare head and neck pain syndromes: a systematic review of the literature. J Neurol 2004; 251(Suppl 1):I19–30.
59. Bogduk N, Govind J. Cervicogenic headache: an assessment of the evidence on clinical diagnosis, invasive tests, and treatment. Lancet Neurol 2009;8(10): 959–68.
60. De Hertogh W, Vaes P, Beckwée D, et al. Lack of impairment of kinaesthetic sensibility in cervicogenic headache patients. Cephalalgia 2008;28:323–8.
61. Fernandez-de-las-Penas C, Alonso-Blanco C, Cuadrado ML, et al. Spinal manipulative therapy in the management of cervicogenic headache. Headache 2005; 45:1260–3.
62. Haas M, Spegman A, Peterson D, et al. Does manipulation for chronic cervicogenic headache: a pilot randomized controlled trial. Spine J 2010;10:117–28.
63. Haldeman S, Dagenais S. Choosing a treatment for cervicogenic headache: when? what? how much? Spine J 2010;10:169–71.

Managing and Treating Tension-type Headache

Frederick Freitag, DO

KEYWORDS

- OnabotulinumtoxinA • Migraine • Tension-type • Anti-depressants

KEY POINTS

- Although tension-type headache is ubiquitous, only a relatively small percentage of the population has these headaches occurring with sufficient frequency and severity to cause them to seek out medical attention.
- Assessment of the headaches includes assessment for other headache disorders that may overlap it, such as a chronic migraine.
- Coexisting diseases that may contribute to the process, such as mood disorders and mechanical disorders of the spine and neck, require investigation.
- Treatment is optimized by appropriate use of acute medications and preventive treatments that may include drugs in the antidepressant classes along with nonpharmacologic modalities and other alternative treatments ranging from biofeedback to manual therapy to the use of botulinum toxin type A injections.

HISTORICAL CONSIDERATIONS

The concept of what constitutes tension-type headache has been undergoing revision for more than 100 years. To a degree this represents continuing evolution of the understanding of this disorder. In past decades tension-type headache was referred to as muscle contraction or muscle tension headache, psychogenic headache, interval headache, and depressive headache. Each of these reflects on components of the headache that individual clinicians believed to represent the causative nature of the headache or its association with other disease states. Muscle contraction headache was used to describe the musculoskeletal quality to the pain and its distribution in the head and neck area. The evolution of describing tension-type headache began in great part with the work of Olesen and coworkers[1] and the methodologic issues that arose in studying treatments for migraine headache in patients with interval headache. In the past 15 years work by Lipton and coworkers[2] examining the treatment of migraine with sumatriptan further led to differentiation of the true tension-type headache from those tension-type headaches or interval headaches occurring in patients with migraine and drawing a possible association between these interval tension-type

Department of Neurosciences, Baylor University Medical Center, 9101 North Central Expressway, Suite 400, Dallas, TX 75231, USA
E-mail address: dhcdoc@gmail.com

Med Clin N Am 97 (2013) 281–292
http://dx.doi.org/10.1016/j.mcna.2012.12.003   medical.theclinics.com
0025-7125/13/$ – see front matter © 2013 Elsevier Inc. All rights reserved.

headache as a mild or early and poorly differentiated form of migraine headache. The most recent version of the International Headache Society diagnostic criteria provides a clearer differentiation between migraine headache and tension-type headache.[3] The International Headache Classification committee criteria for tension-type headache have undergone changes since its first publication. New clinical and basic research data have led to these revisions and practical division based on potential impact. Overall, tension-type headache remains the most common of headache disorders and is estimated by the Classification committee as afflicting up to 78% of the world population. Differentiation between infrequent and frequent episodic tension-type headache is based on frequency but also reflects potential impact of the disorder (**Table 1**).

Although pericranial muscle tenderness may occur with these disorders this is more closely associated with the episodic forms because there is suggestion that the chronic form of the disorder may represent a more central pain disorder. Overlapping characteristics is a possibly with chronic migraine in some patients rendering diagnosis challenging.

Although the pain is typically localized to the scalp, variations on this are not uncommon and may present with neck pain, neck stiffness or limitation of movement, or pain with chewing. In patients with chronic tension-type headache it is not unusual to see complaints of pain that is more than mild to moderate intensity. In the older terminology this increased pain intensity, which may be rated at maximal levels of severity, would have been associated with psychogenic or depressive headache.

PATHOPHYSIOLOGY

Involvement of the pericranial muscles in these chronic tension-type headaches may be associated with pain or may be found with chronic spasticity of the muscles without associated palpatory tenderness. Diamond and Dalessio[4] postulated a multistep process contributing to the involvement of the pericranial and cervical muscles in tension-type headache. They suggested that local factors in the muscle tissue could

Table 1 Criteria for tension-type headache			
	Infrequent Episodic Tension-Type Headache	**Frequent Episodic Tension-Type Headache**	**Chronic Tension-Type Headache**
Frequency	<1/mo	1–14 d/mo	≥15 d/mo over ≥3 mo
Impact	None	Little	May be significant
Duration	Minutes to days	Minutes to days	Days to constant
IHC-2 criteria	2 of 4 of: Bilateral Nonpulsatile Mild or moderate pain intensity No exacerbation by routine physical activity	2 of 4 of: Bilateral Nonpulsatile Mild or moderate pain intensity No exacerbation by routine physical activity	2 of 4 of: Bilateral Nonpulsatile Mild or moderate pain intensity No exacerbation by routine physical activity
IHC-2 associated symptom criteria	No anorexia, nausea, or vomiting May have photophobia or phonophobia	Anorexia, but no nausea or vomiting May have photophobia or phonophobia	May have mild nausea or may have photophobia or phonophobia but not any two

Abbreviation: IHC, International Headache Classification.

provoke a local neural impulse initiating a reflex response at the spinal cord level leading to muscle contraction but also to a polysynaptic relay of the stimulus to thalamic and cortical levels. They postulated that brain activates the reticulospinal system sending impulses through this efferent tract to the gamma efferent fibers at the spinal cord level causing activation of the muscle spindle leading to a monosynaptic reflex through the ventral cord to efferent peripheral nerve augmenting the muscle contraction. In the absence of blocking factors the increased muscle tone would lead to inhibition of the muscle spindle. If local factors continue to elicit activation of the afferent paths or if changes in cortical activity promote reticulospinal efferent transmission the muscle fibers would experience increasing muscle tone to the point of spasm and associated pain.

Postural mechanical factors involving the cervical spine may also be present in patients with tension-type headache with pericranial muscle involvement. This may involve trigger point acuity, restriction of motion, and anterior head positioning as contributors to the occurrence of more chronic headache.[5] Underlying disk disease or degenerative joint disease of the apophyseal joints of the cervical spine may lead to increased localized muscle spasm and pain. Chronically, patterns of altered cervical mechanics may occur furthering the cervical contribution to the headache process. The structure of the neck musculature, with muscles overlapping not only single but several cervical segments, in addition to the long muscles of the neck and the trapezius muscle may serve as distant initiating factors associated with muscle spasm and pain referred to higher cervical levels. Elements of cervical dystonia may also be found in this group of patients with chronic tension-type headache. Typically the amount of dystonia present is quite minimal and may be reflected by a slight tilt of the head toward the side of the dystonia. Involvement of muscles in the anterior and lateral neck is typically associated with this pattern of pericranial muscle involvement.

Referral of head pain from upper cervical structures is made possible by convergence of cervical and trigeminal nociceptive afferent information in the trigeminocervical nucleus. Upper cervical segmental and C2-3 zygapophysial joint dysfunction is recognized as a potential source of afferent input in patients with the primary headache disorders of migraine, cluster, and tension-type headaches. Furthermore, referral of head pain has been demonstrated from symptomatic upper cervical segments and the C2-3 zygapophysial joints, suggesting that head pain referral may be a characteristic of cervical afferent involvement in headache. A recent study[6] examining this found that manual techniques to these upper cervical segments reproduced the type of headache pain experienced by patients with migraine and tension-type headache but did not lead to headache pain in the control population.

Biologically, tension-type headache differs from migraine with such factors as biologic peptides. Several studies have examined calcitonin gene–related peptide,[7] substance P,[8] neuropeptide Y, and vasoactive intestinal peptide. These peptides do not change during pain versus pain-free times, nor do they differ from a control non-headache population. The serum levels of N-acetylaspartate[9] may be considered a useful marker of neuronal functioning. Levels of this substance are significantly reduced in patients with various forms of migraine compared with episodic and chronic tension-type headache and the control population.

EPIDEMIOLOGY

A study by Schwartz and coworkers[10] estimated the overall prevalence of episodic tension-type headache at the following:

- 38.3% of the population
- Females age 30–39 years, approximately 47%

- African-American descent overall, 22.8%
- Increased with increasing levels of education
- Graduate school level education, approximately 50%

By contrast, chronic tension-type headache had a far lower prevalence of about 2%. Women were more likely than men to experience the chronic form of the disorder.[11] Although the relationship of menstruation to migraine is well established, a recent study showed that women with tension-type headache were twice as likely as women with migraine to have their headache occur only with menses. These headaches associated with the menses were also associated with higher levels of disability on the MIDAS score than those headaches not associated with menses. The prevalence declined with increasing education compared with the increase seen with the episodic form. Although one expects episodic tension-type headache to have little impact on function, Schwartz and coworkers[10] found that 8.3% of individuals lost days from work and nearly half worked at decreased levels of effectiveness. Those with the chronic form were more highly impacted, with one-fifth of patients missing work.

CLINICAL EXAMINATION

Physical examination findings are generally absent or minimal in the episodic varieties of tension-type headache. Tenderness of palpation or palpatory muscle spasm may be present if there is involvement of distinct muscle groups in the head and neck region. In patients with chronic tension-type headache, where there is no involvement of the pericranial muscles, a normal examination is the rule. The potential central nature of the pain of chronic tension-type headache may account for the absence of positive findings on examination in the presence of significant levels of pain.

DIAGNOSTIC TESTING

In the primary headache disorder, such as migraine and tension-type headache, the incidence of abnormal radiologic findings in patients with a normal physical and neurologic examination is rare[12] or even nonexistent, as may be the case in tension-type headache. Despite this neuroimaging should be considered in the patient with a normal neurologic examination if the headaches are rapidly increasing in frequency, poorly responsive to simple analgesics, or associated with new or atypical neurologic symptoms. Plain skull radiographs may be helpful in the elderly patient with a new onset of headache to examine for Paget disease. Plain radiographs of the cervical spine or magnetic resonance imaging of the cervical spine can be helpful in evaluating for concomitant conditions that might influence or cause tension-type headache.

Baseline chemistries and blood counts should be considered in the evaluation especially if the patient will be taking daily preventive medications. This should include thyroid evaluation, because hypothyroidism can present with a headache resembling that of tension-type headache.

The role of personality traits and psychological disorders has long been associated with tension-type headache. The Akershus study[13] of chronic headache demonstrated that patients with chronic tension-type headaches were more likely to experience a high level of neuroticism and psychological distress than the general population. The authors raise the interesting query for further study of assessing these psychological markers as cause or effect in tension-type headache.

In patients where psychiatric comorbidity[14] is present the use of appropriate assessment by a psychologist and screening psychological questionnaire should be considered.

DIFFERENTIAL DIAGNOSIS

Perhaps the area that is most challenging in the patient with tension-type headache is differentiating tension-type headache from migraine headache. This becomes more problematic with daily and near daily headache where there is more likely to be similarities to the patient with chronic migraine.

Chronic migraine is a complication of frequent episodic migraine headache or other complicating issues presenting as a daily or near daily pattern of headache. In the past this phenomenon has been known as migraine with tension-type headache, mixed headache, combined headache, migraine with interval headache, transformed migraine, and chronic daily headache.

Migraine by definition is typically a moderate or severe headache attack that may be unilateral and may have an exacerbation by physical activity, with the pain having to it a throbbing or pulsatile component. Normally the attacks have well-defined beginning and ending points with duration of headache of between 4 and 72 hours. During the attack patients have nausea or vomiting, or photophobia and phonophobia. These symptoms occur if the attack is permitted to go to maximal intensity of pain without successful treatment. Intervention by the patient even with medication that is not capable of fully alleviating the migraine may blunt the intensity of the associated symptoms and characteristics of the headache or alleviate entire components. This intervention and the failure to obtain this information in the headache history is perhaps the most common reason for migraine and tension-type headache to be misdiagnosed. The alleviation or blunting of the migraine symptoms can readily make the migraine attack seem as a tension-type headache. Migraine and tension-type headache are associated with trigger factors that may elicit the occurrence of headache. These trigger factors are very similar between the two disorders.[15] With overlap of trigger factors, especially if these are of a psychological nature, such as stress, the physician may be even more likely to attribute the headache as a tension-type headache rather than migraine.

In the evaluation of the patient with possible tension-type headache, it is important to assess for several key factors. First, whether the patient has a history of migraine headaches. If they have this in their history then tracking any changes in the migraine pattern may lead to a diagnosis of chronic migraine rather than chronic tension-type headache. Second, it is necessary to know if the attacks of headache that the patient is describing are treated or untreated headaches. If they are untreated and fail to meet criteria for migraine then the diagnosis of tension-type headache is likely. If the attacks the patient describes are treated attacks then it is best to obtain information on any attacks the patient may have had, but that were left untreated. This second query is of importance in the patient whose headaches remain episodic, because the partially treated episodic migraine without aura may seem to be a tension-type headache. A third factor to consider, more in differentiating episodic tension-type headache from the chronic variety, relates to the overuse of medications for acute treatment. Just as may occur in the patient with migraine, so too in the tension-type headache, the overuse of acute medications may cloud the true diagnosis, because only after the patient has been free of medication overuse for at least 3 months can the diagnosis be established with certainty.

The nasal sinus regions may lead to headache with episodic infection and chronic disorders of the sinuses. Overlap syndromes with migraine and tension-type headache may occur in these patients and require an appropriate examination of the nasal passages and if necessary computed tomography scan without contrast using coronal sections to establish the diagnosis. The absence of abnormal findings on examination or on scanning helps to alleviate the nasal sinuses areas as a cause of the pain. On examination of the nasal passage the patient with headache from this origin is expected to have mucopurelent discharge and evidence of contact between the nasal septum and the turbinates. Computed tomography scan findings reflect acute infection with significant air fluid levels or complete obliteration of the sinus cavities by fluid. In an interesting experiment, Wolff[16] demonstrated that it required pressure of 200 mm Hg rising steadily over time to elicit pain from the maxillary sinuses and that sustained pressure over several hours of 150 to 180 mm Hg was needed to elicit even the sensation of pressure from the maxillary sinus cavity. Similarly, pain from engorgement of the nasal turbinates did not occur until these pressures had been achieved and maintained for several hours.

Pain in the temporalis muscle, which extends over the temperomandibular joint to attach to the mandible, may be a source of pain in tension-type headache. Because of the effects of sustained contraction of this muscle on the temporomandibular joint there may be pain specifically elicited from this joint associated with tension-type headache. Differentiation from temporomandibular joint syndrome is necessary.

TREATMENT CONSIDERATIONS

Treatment of tension-type headache may involve pharmacotherapeutic agents and other approaches. The pharmacotherapy of tension headache includes medications for acute treatment and medications for the chronic form of tension-type headache for preventative treatment. The other approaches to tension-type headache may include behavioral approaches, such as counseling and biofeedback; physical methods including physical therapy; manipulative treatments; and injection techniques.

The acute medications for tension-type headache are primarily directed for use as analgesic relief of the pain (**Table 2**). Muscle relaxant agents are used as episodic acute treatments and as part of preventive treatment.

Because the pain of tension-type headache is mild to moderate in intensity for most patients, the use of opioids is avoided in this headache disorder except for isolated headaches in patients who are well known to the treating clinician. Patients with chronic tension-type headache with their daily or near daily headaches are susceptible to becoming dependent on opioids if they become a primary pain medication.

Simple analgesics are the starting point for treating tension-type headache acutely. Acetaminophen, aspirin, and over-the-counter nonsteroidal anti-inflammatory drugs (NSAIDS) provide effective relief clinically. Because daily excessive use of even these agents may be linked to medication overuse headache, patients should be counseled in their appropriate use to avoid these sequelae. Combination analgesic agents with caffeine have proved effective in clinical trials.[17,18] From our study,[18] caffeine may not serve as an adjunct in pain relief but may contribute a portion of the analgesic activity.

The NSAIDS at over-the-counter and at prescription strengths have been demonstrated to be useful in tension-type headache. A recent meta-analysis[19] demonstrated that low-strength NSAIDS were comparable with acetaminophen with comparable adverse event risks. Higher strengths of the NSAIDS proved to be more efficacious than acetaminophen but with a somewhat higher chance of adverse events. The choice of which of these analgesic agents and the strength of the preparation involve weighing the potential benefit versus risk and personal preference and individual response.

There are varieties of skeletal muscle relaxants and antispasticity agents that find their way into treatment of tension-type headache. Unfortunately, the use of these is

Table 2
Guidelines for use of selected abortive therapies in the treatment of tension-type headache

Medication	Dose/Route/Clarification
NSAIDs	Major side effects are GI-related
Acetylsalicylic acid	650 mg (2 regular-strength tablets) stat (po)
Celecoxib	200–400 mg
Diclofenac	12.5–100 mg (po)
Diflunisal	500 mg q 8–12 h
Etodolac	200–400 mg q 6–8 h
Fenoprofen	300–600 mg tid-qid
Flurbiprofen	100 mg stat, repeat in 1 h (po)
Ibuprofen	400–600 mg q 6 h (po)
Ketoprofen	100 mg stat, then 50 mg if needed in 1 h
Ketorolac	60 mg (IM); limit use to 1 dose
Meclofenamate	200 mg stat, repeat x 1 after 1 h (po)
Mefenamic acid	50 mg q 4–6 h prn
Naproxen sodium	550 mg stat, then 275 mg in 1 h (po)
Tolmetin	200–600 mg tid prn
Muscle relaxants with/without analgesics	
Baclofen	5–20 mg tid-qid (po); do not abruptly discontinue drug
Carisoprodol	350 mg tid (po); short-term use only, habit-forming; subject to abuse by users of illicit drugs
Carisoprodol 200 mg and aspirin 325 mg	1 tablet tid (po); short-term use only, habit-forming; subject to abuse by users of illicit drugs
Chlorzoxazone	500 mg qid
Cyclobenzaprine	10 mg bid (po)
Metaxalone	800 mg (2 tablets) tid-qid (po)
Methocarbamol	800 mg (2 tablets) tid-qid (po)
Orphenadrine citrate	100 mg bid (po)
Orphenadrine citrate 50 mg, aspirin 770 mg, and caffeine 60 mg	1 tablet bid-tid (po)
Tizanidine	2 mg qid

Abbreviations: GI, gastrointestinal; IM, intramuscularly.

merely anecdotal because there are no well-defined controlled trials of them in tension-type headache.

In those with frequent headache requiring acute treatments or where there is impact of headache on functional ability an attempt to induce a remission of these headaches, such as with the use of daily preventive medications, may be in order. Although several of the long-duration antispaciticity agents, such as baclofen or tizanidine, may be of benefit, the mainstay of preventive treatment in tension-type headache is the antidepressant medications.[20] Again, there is a paucity of well-controlled trials with these agents to support their use, much of the literature on it being intermixed with chronic daily headache, which included patients with chronic migraine among other diagnoses. Practically, however, it is these agents that are most likely to afford relief from the chronic recurrent headaches regardless of the etiologic issues underlying their cause. The antidepressants fall into three major groups: (1) the tricyclic antidepressants (TCA), (2) the monoamine oxidase inhibitors, and (3) the serotonin-specific reuptake inhibitors and the norepinephrine/serotonin-reuptake inhibitors and other novel antidepressants. The TCA group has the best clinical efficacy for tension-type headache. This may be the result of the breadth of pharmacologic activity they have, which may produce a direct analgesic effect as part of that mechanism.

The range of pharmacologic effects of TCAs (**Table 3**) needs to be appreciated for optimal selection of an agent based on the patient's tolerance of medications, coexisting illnesses, associated mood disorders, and sleep habits. Typically, it is wise to inquire whether a patient has a concomitant sleep disorder. Patients with insomnia usually fare best with a sedating TCA with or without a mild benzodiazepine to initiate sleep. Those with chronic fatigue and daytime tiredness tolerate a TCA like protryptiline far better. The anticholinergic effects contribute to the dry mouth, constipation, and blurred vision that patients may have as adverse events. Reducing the relative effects here may be helpful for those who cannot acclimate to them. The sedative effects are linked in part to the antihistaminic effects of these drugs. This antihistaminic inhibition effect may also contribute to carbohydrate cravings and weight gain and couple with the anticholinergic activity to affect cognitive issues adversely.

The monoamine oxidase inhibitors are not commonly used outside of specialty clinics because of the issues related to drug interactions, dietary restrictions, and the potential for serious adverse events to occur with these interactions. However, in refractive patients who have failed to achieve benefit with more traditional therapies they have proved exceptional for their efficacy.[21]

The newer antidepressants have been used in treating chronic daily headache but again much of this use has been in patients with chronic migraine or combination of headache disorders. However, they possess comparatively exceptional tolerability compared with the TCAs. The European guidelines[22] support the use of the TCA amitriptyline and two newer agents having effects on serotonin and norepinephrine, receptors, venlafaxine and mirtazipine.

Imipramine, one of the TCA class antidepressants, was compared with transcutaneous electrical nerve stimulation as a treatment of tension-type headache.[23] As expected from clinical practice the imipramine group showed substantial headache

Table 3
Antidepressants and receptor affinity

Drug	Serotonin Inhibition	Norepinephrine Inhibition	Dopamine Inhibition	Sedative Effects	Anticholinergic Effects	Histamine Inhibitions
Amitriptyline	Moderate	Weak	Inactive	Strong	Strong	Moderate
Doxepin	Moderate	Moderate	Inactive	Strong	Strong	Strong
Nortriptyline	Weak	Fairly potent	Inactive	Mild	Moderate	Mild
Imipramine	Fairly potent	Moderate	Inactive	Moderate	Strong	Mild
Protryptiline	Weak	Fairly potent	Inactive	None	Strong	None
Desipramine	Weak	Potent	Inactive	Mild	Moderate	Mild or none
Trimipramine	Weak	Weak	Inactive	Moderate	Moderate	Moderate
Amoxapine	Weak	Potent	Moderate	Mild	Mild	Mild
Maprotiline	Weak	Moderate	Inactive	Moderate	Moderate	Moderate

reduction compared with baseline. Similarly, transcutaneous electrical nerve stimulation also led to improvement compared with baseline but to a statistically lesser degree than imipramine. Perhaps one factor that may enter into the differential response between treatments is patient preference[24] as demonstrated in a trial where patients could elect treatment with amitriptyline or hypnotic relaxation, in which those who choose the hypnotic relaxation had superior outcomes to a standard dose of amitriptyline.

A novel therapeutic approach using memantine, an N-methyl-D-aspartate antagonist, which would work on central pain mechanisms in chronic tension-type headache, has been studied.[25] Although it failed to produce a statistically significant difference from placebo in this small study, the results were encouraging with side effects mostly of nausea and dizziness.

Of the nonpharmacologic techniques for tension-type headache the preferred approach based on efficacy is the combination of biofeedback along with cognitive behavioral counseling.[26] These techniques focus on not just the stress issues that may contribute to the headaches, but also on the muscle relaxation training in biofeedback to offer a specific method to help reduce the pain of associated headaches. In the training for biofeedback the patient has surface electrodes attached to the scalp, face, or neck region of pain to register the amount of muscle activity occurring. Through guided exercises patients learn to control the underlying muscle tension and help to alleviate the headache. The technique require a combination of hands-on training with a therapist experienced in its use along with regular at home practice sessions.

Massage and physical therapy have been examined in the treatment of tension-type headache. Although there may be specific patients who have postural mechanical factors at play in their headaches who benefit from these treatments, the techniques in general produce little in the way of positive benefits. Manual therapies performed by a chiropractor or osteopathic physician have also been studied in the treatment of tension-type headache. The results have been mixed. Some studies reporting significant benefit, others little if any. Many issues have clouded these results including diagnosis of the headaches being treated, the techniques used, and the choice of masking or alternative active controls for assessment of outcome of these studies. Proper assessment of the patient for alterations in muscle tone and postural and mechanical effects may, coupled with appropriate and comprehensive diagnosis, lead to successful treatment with these techniques.

Acupuncture, which has a long history of use and effectiveness in treatment of pain, has been subjected to study in the treatment of tension-type headache. A review and analysis of some 120 studies of its use suggested that variability in the nature of the trials diminished the potential for optimal clarity of this ancient method.[27] The meta-analysis suggested that sham treatment was as effective as real acupuncture. Further review of the 43 studies that lent themselves to comparative review found electro-acupuncture to be more efficacious than manual acupuncture; needle retention with 30 minutes being better than no needle retention; and twice-a-week treatment was better than once-a-week treatment. This study supports the use of acupuncture in the preventive treatment of tension-type headache with specific caveats for improving efficacy.

The use of injections, such as trigger pointing, is covered elsewhere in this issue. For patients with localized areas of muscle pain and tenderness these may have use as part of a comprehensive treatment program. Specific techniques to address tension-type headache have been examined with the use of botulinum toxin A. The trials have been small and lacking in solid control groups, but have suggested that there are some patients who benefit from the injections.[28,29] Those with pericranial muscle tenderness may be more likely to respond.[30] The mechanism by which botulinum toxin A exerts its effects in tension-type headache may be by direct effects at the neuromuscular junction and by potential central effects that may modulate the pain tracks centrally. The choice of injections sites is typical guided by the patient's areas of pain and associated muscle spasm. It is important to assess the mechanics that may contribute to the pain. For example, minimal cervical dystonia may occur involving the sternocleidomastoid muscle. The chronic shortening of the muscle may not be painful but the pull exerted on the posterior muscles on the opposite side of the neck may be the source of the pain. Injecting into the area of pain fails to alleviate the problem and may intensify the situation in some patients, whereas injection into the affected sternocleidomastoid muscle produces relaxation of the spasticity and relief of the pain on the posterior opposite side of the neck. Repetitive injections with botulinum toxin may be required to demonstrate an adequate response. There may be a high rate of placebo response with the initial series of injections or the results may be minimal or brief. Repeating the injections minimizes placebo effects and may demonstrate more robust relief of the headaches and expanding duration of relief from the headaches and neck pain. Side effects tend to be negligible for most patients beyond the initial discomfort of the injections. Cost may be prohibitive for many patients because its use in headache has not been approved by the Food and Drug Administration in chronic tension-type headache compared with chronic migraine, where it is well accepted as an effective therapeutic agent.

SUMMARY

Although tension-type headache is ubiquitous, only a relatively small percentage of the population has these headaches occurring with sufficient frequency and severity to cause them to seek out medical attention. This small group, however, may have substantial impact from their disease on productivity and quality of life. Assessment of the headaches includes assessment for other headache disorders that may overlap it, such as a chronic migraine. Additionally, coexisting diseases that may contribute to the process, such as mood disorders and mechanical disorders of the spine and neck, require investigation. Treatment is optimized by appropriate use of acute medications and preventive treatments that may include drugs in the antidepressant classes along with nonpharmacologic modalities and other alternative treatments ranging from biofeedback to manual therapy to the use of botulinum toxin type A injections.

REFERENCES

1. Olesen J, Krabbe AA, Tfelt-Hansen P. Methodological aspects of prophylactic drug trials in migraine. Cephalalgia 1981;1:127–41.
2. Lipton RB, Cady RK, Stewart WF, et al. Diagnostic lessons from the spectrum study. Neurology 2002;58(9 Suppl 6):S27–31.
3. Headache Classification Subcommittee of The International Headache Society. The international classification of headache disorders, 2nd edition. Cephalalgia 2004;24(Suppl 1):50–60.
4. Diamond S, Dalessio DJ. Muscle contraction headache. In: Diamond D, Dalessio DJ, editors. The practicing physician's approach to headache. 4th edition. Baltimore (MD): Williams and Wilkins; 1986. p. 99–113.
5. Sohn JH, Choi HC, Lee SM, et al. Differences in cervical musculoskeletal impairment between episodic and chronic tension-type headache. Cephalalgia 2010; 30(12):1514–23.

6. Watson DH, Drummond PD. Head pain referral during examination of the neck in migraine and tension-type headache. Headache 2012;52(8):1226–35.
7. Ashina M, Bendtsen L, Jensen R, et al. Plasma levels of calcitonin-gene related peptide in chronic tension type headache. Neurology 2000;55:1335–40.
8. Ashina M, Bendtsen L, Jensen R, et al. Plasma levels of substance P, neuropeptides Y and vasoactive intestinal peptide in patients with chronic tension type headache. Pain 1999;83:541–7.
9. de Tommaso M, Ceci E, Pica C, et al. Serum levels of N-acetyl-aspartate in migraine and tension-type headache. J Headache Pain 2012;13(5):389–94.
10. Schwartz BS, Stewart WF, Simon D, et al. Epidemiology of tension type headache. JAMA 1998;279:381–3.
11. Karli N, Baykan B, Ertaş M, et al, Turkish Headache Prevalence Study Group. Impact of sex hormonal changes on tension-type headache and migraine: a cross-sectional population-based survey in 2,600 women. J Headache Pain 2012;13(7):557–65.
12. Silberstein S. Practice Parameter: Evidence-based guidelines for migraine headache (an evidence based review): Report of the Quality Standards Subcommittee of the American Academy of Neurology. Neurology 2000;55:754–65.
13. Aaseth K, Grande RB, Leiknes KA, et al. Personality traits and psychological distress in persons with chronic tension-type headache. The Akershus study of chronic headache. Acta Neurol Scand 2011;124(6):375–82.
14. London LH, Shulman B, Diamond S. The role of psychometric testing and psychological treatment in tension type headache. Curr Pain Headache Rep 2001;5:467–71.
15. Haque DB, Rahman DK, Hoque DA, et al. Precipitating and relieving factors of migraine versus tension type headache. BMC Neurol 2012;12(1):82.
16. Wolff HG. Muscle of the head and neck as sources of headache and other pain. In: Wolff HG, editor. Headache and other head pain. New York: Oxford University Press; 1948. p. 456–9.
17. Rabello GD, Forte LV, Galvao AC. Clinical evaluation of the efficacy of the paracetamol and caffeine combination in the treatment of tension headache. Arq Neuropsiquiatr 2000;58:90–8.
18. Diamond S, Balm TK, Freitag FG. Ibuprofen plus caffeine in the treatment of tension-type headache. Clin Pharmacol Ther 2000;68:312–9.
19. Yoon YJ, Kim JH, Kim SY, et al. A comparison of efficacy and safety of nonsteroidal anti-inflammatory drugs versus acetaminophen in the treatment of episodic tension-type headache: a meta-analysis of randomized placebo-controlled trial studies. Korean J Fam Med 2012;33(5):262–71.
20. Holyroyd KA, O'Donnell FJ, Stensland M, et al. Management of chronic tension type headache with tricyclic antidepressants medication, stress management therapy, and their combination: a randomized controlled trial. JAMA 2001;285:2208–15.
21. Freitag FG, Diamond S, Solomon GD. Antidepressants and the treatment of mixed headache: MAO inhibitors and combined use of MAO inhibitors and tricyclic antidepressants in the recidivist headache patient. In: Rose FC, editor. Advances in headache research. London: John Libbey & Co. Ltd.; 1987. p. 271–5.
22. Bendtsen L, Evers S, Linde M, et al. EFNS guideline on the treatment of tension-type headache: report of an EFNS task force. Eur J Neurol 2010;17(11):1318–25.
23. Mousavi SA, Mirbod SM, Khorvash F. Comparison between efficacy of imipramine and transcutaneous electrical nerve stimulation in the prophylaxis of chronic tension-type headache: a randomized controlled clinical trial. J Res Med Sci 2011;16(7):923–7.

24. Ezra Y, Gotkine M, Goldman S, et al. Hypnotic relaxation vs amitriptyline for tension-type headache: let the patient choose. Headache 2012;52(5):785–91.
25. Lindelof K, Bendtsen L. Memantine for prophylaxis of chronic tension-type headache: a double-blind, randomized, crossover clinical trial. Cephalalgia 2009; 29(3):314–21.
26. Andrasik F. Behavioral treatment approaches to chronic headache. Neurol Sci 2003;24(Suppl 2):S80–5.
27. Hao XA, Xue CC, Dong L, et al. Factors associated with conflicting findings on acupuncture for tension-type headache: qualitative and quantitative analyses. J Altern Complement Med 2012. [Epub ahead of print].
28. Freitag FG. Preventative treatment for migraine and tension-type headaches; do drugs having effects on muscle spasm and tone have a role? CNS Drugs 2003; 17(6):373–81.
29. Gobel H, Heinze A, Heinze-Kuhn K, et al. Evidenced based medicine: botulinum toxin A in migraine and tension type headache. J Neurol 2001;248(Suppl 1):34–8.
30. Karadaş O, Ipekdal IH, Ulaş UH, et al. Botulinum neuro-toxin type-A in the treatment of chronic tension type headache associated with pericranial tenderness. Agri 2012;24(1):9–14.

Pain of Ocular and Periocular Origin

Corey W. Waldman, MD[a], Steven D. Waldman, MD, JD[b,*],
Reid A. Waldman[b]

KEYWORDS

- Corneal abrasion • Hordeolum • Uveitis • Scleritis • Cluster headache
- Optic neuritis

KEY POINTS

- Most diseases of the eye and periocular regions that cause blindness are relatively painless.
- The rich innervation of the cornea, conjunctiva, and periocular region means that even minor problems such as a superficial corneal abrasion can result in severe pain that is completely out of proportion to the scope and risk of the pathologic abnormality.
- Glaucoma is one of the leading causes of blindness in the world.
- Referred eye pain is common because the eye shares innervation by the first division of the trigeminal nerve with many other structures in the head.

Headache pain of ocular and periocular origin represents a special challenge to the clinician. Pain in this anatomic region is unique because (1) most diseases of the eye and periocular regions that cause blindness are relatively painless; yet the fear of blindness is ever present in any patient with eye pain; (2) most painful conditions of the eye and periocular region associated with headache do not cause blindness in spite of the aforementioned fear to the contrary; (3) both laypersons and most health care professionals approach any problem involving the eye with great fear and trepidation because of the potential for disastrous consequences if a mistake in diagnosis or treatment is made; (4) the rich innervation of the cornea, conjunctiva, and periocular region means that even minor problems such as a superficial corneal abrasion can result in severe pain that is completely out of proportion to the scope and risk of the injury; and (5) if the pathologic process responsible for the patient's pain resides in the eye, an ophthalmologist is needed, and if it does not involve the eye, the ophthalmologist has little to offer, thus leaving the clinician to sort out the cause and provide the treatment for the patient's pain.

Large portions of this text were originally published in Waldman SD and Waldman CW. Pain of Ocular and Periocular Origin. In: Waldman SD, editor. Pain Management. 2nd Edition. Chapter 53: Elsevier; 2011. p. 482–93.
[a] Krieger Eye Institute At Sinai, 2411 West Belvedere Avenue, Baltimore, USA; [b] School of Medicine, University of Missouri-Kansas City, 2411 Holmes, Kansas City, Missouri, MO 64108, USA
* Corresponding author.
E-mail address: sdwaldmanmd@gmail.com

Med Clin N Am 97 (2013) 293–307
http://dx.doi.org/10.1016/j.mcna.2012.12.004
0025-7125/13/$ – see front matter © 2013 Elsevier Inc. All rights reserved.

Further complicating the issue is an interesting diagnostic conundrum unique to patients suffering from ocular or periocular pain. The conundrum finds its basis in the fact that, although the clinician, ophthalmologist, and, for that matter, the patient can easily identify "the red eye" (ie, the eye that is obviously inflamed, infected, or traumatized), yet the patient and even the skilled nonophthalmologist will often completely miss the findings of serious vision-threatening disease in what is known in the ophthalmologic literature as the "quiet eye." The identification of these hidden findings within the "quiet eye" requires a careful ophthalmologic examination that is well beyond the expertise of the nonophthalmologist. **Box 1** presents a list of some of the more common ocular or periocular diseases that may reside within the "quiet eye." Thus, the care of such patients is more challenging in comparison with patients with less-threatening painful conditions, such as low back pain. That said, as a practical matter, the management of most patients with headache pain thought to be of ocular and periocular origin is relatively straightforward. Primary diseases of the eye are best treated by an ophthalmologist and the clinician's role in this setting is to attempt to identify those patients with primary eye and periocular disease responsible for the patient's pain symptoms and refer them in a timely manner to the ophthalmologist for definitive treatment of the ocular pathologic process responsible for the pain. For those patients with ocular and periocular pain that is unrelated to primary eye disease, identification and treatment of the painful condition usually become the responsibility of the clinician.

THE SENSORY INNERVATION OF THE EYE

The primary sensory innervation of the eye is mediated via the trigeminal ganglion.[1] The first division of the trigeminal nerve (V_1 ophthalmic division) carries the bulk of the pain impulses from the eye itself via the long ciliary branches of the nasociliary nerve (**Fig. 1**). The infratrochlear branch of the nasociliary nerve also provides sensory innervation to the medial portion of the eyelids, the adjacent nose, and the lacrimal sac. Trigeminal fibers intimately associated with the intraorbital parasympathetic ganglion and its parasympathetic fibers and the second cervical ganglion and its postganglionic sympathetic fibers may also subserve ocular and periocular pain. Other branches of the first division of the trigeminal nerve, the frontal and lacrimal nerves, provide sensory

---

Box 1
Painful ocular and periocular diseases that may hide within the quiet eye

- Glaucoma
- Uveitis
- Optic neuropathy
- Optic neuritis
- Intraocular neoplasm
- Orbital neoplasm
- Scleritis of the posterior globe
- Corneal pathology
- Foreign bodies
- Infections in immunocompromised hosts
- Inflammation of the extraocular muscles
- Granulomatous disease of the orbit

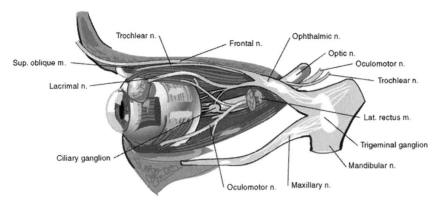

Fig. 1. The sensory innervation of the eye. (*From* Waldman SD. Pain management. 2nd edition. Elsevier; 2011. Figure 53-1.)

innervation to the upper eyelid, forehead, and the frontal sinus and the lacrimal gland and portions of the conjunctiva, respectively. Numerous fibers from the sphenopalatine ganglion also interact with trigeminal somatic fibers and the sympathetic and parasympathetic ganglia and trigeminal somatic fibers and may serve an important role in some painful conditions that involve the eye, such as Sluder neuralgia and cluster headache. The second division of the trigeminal nerve (V_2 maxillary) provides sensory innervation to the lower eyelid and conjunctiva via the infraorbital nerve.

Interestingly, the cornea receives most of the sensory innervation of the eye, with the density of sensory innervation of the cornea rivaled only by that of the anal mucosa.[2] Teleologically, this density of sensory innervation presumably serves to enhance the mechanisms to protect the most important sense organ by allowing the blink response and the convergence avoidance reflex to protect the eye.

In addition to the dense concentration of pain receptors to transmit the afferent sensation of pain via the trigeminal ganglion to higher centers, thermal receptors for cold and heat are also found throughout the eye. These mechanoreceptors are found in both the cornea and the iris and may be responsible for afferent traffic carried via the trigeminal system that may be perceived by the patient as ocular pain even when no actual ocular tissue damage has occurred. Stretching of the extraocular muscles and the dural covering of the optic nerve by mass or tumor may also result in a sensation of ocular pain, even in the absence of actual nerve damage.

COMMON CAUSES OF OCULAR PAIN

The patient with eye pain often presents in an anxious state armed with a detailed history of symptoms. The clinician should begin the evaluation of such patients first by offering reassurance and a calm demeanor and second by rapidly assessing whether the clinical condition presents immediate risk to the patient's vision so that immediate ophthalmologic referral can be undertaken. A targeted history and physical examination will simplify this process (**Box 2**). **Boxes 3** and **4** provide a list of signs and symptoms that should prompt the clinician to consider strongly ophthalmologic referral on an urgent basis.

Styes (Hordeolums)

Styes, or hordeolums, are a common cause of eye pain encountered in clinical practice.[3] More than 98% of styes are caused by *Staphylococcus aureus*.[4] These pus-filled

---

Box 2
The targeted history in patients with headaches attributed to the eye or periocular region

- Is the onset of pain acute or chronic?
- Is the pain associated with any visual loss?
- Is the pain associated with any change in color vision?
- Is the pain associated with any change in visual field?
- Do you experience double vision?
- Do you experience excessive tearing?
- If there is excessive tearing, is it transient or permanent?
- Do you have dry eyes?
- If there is any change in vision, is it transient or permanent?
- If transient, what is the frequency of visual disturbance?
- Is the pain transient or permanent?
- If the pain is transient, what is its frequency?
- If the pain is transient, what is the onset-to peak?
- Is there any fever associated with the pain?
- Are there any systemic symptoms associated with the pain?
- Is there any nausea or vomiting associated with the pain?
- Are there any alterations in smell or hearing associated with the pain?
- Is there jaw pain when chewing food?
- Where is the pain located?
- Does the location of the pain move?
- Is the pain made worse with bright light?
- Is the pain better in darkness?
- Is the pain made worse with eye movement?
- Is the pain throbbing in nature?
- Is the pain shocklike in nature?
- Is the pain pressure or bandlike in nature?
- What is the severity of the pain?

---

abscesses can appear quite suddenly and can run the gamut from small self-limited infections that produce little pain and resolve on their own to rapidly growing, extremely painful abscesses that require immediate surgical incision and drainage and systemic antibiotics for resolution.[4] If the condition is identified early, the use of non–neomycin-containing antibiotic ointment, such as gentamicin or polymyxin-B, and bacitracin ophthalmic ointment combined with frequent applications of warm moist packs usually resolve the problem.[4] If fever is present or the stye does not drain with conservative therapy, systemic antibiotics and immediate ophthalmologic referral for surgical incision and drainage is indicated.[5] If untreated, what begins as a simple localized folliculitis or meibomianitis can evolve into a vision-threatening and life-threatening periorbital cellulitis that has the potential to spread to the adjacent central nervous system.[6]

Box 3
Factors that cause concern in the patient with ocular or periocular pain

Pain associated with fever

Pain associated with systemic illness

History of recent ocular or periocular trauma

Ocular surgery within 60 days

New visual acuity loss

New change in color vision

New visual field defects

Corneal cloudiness or opacification

Anisocoria

Nonreactive pupil

Proptosis

Ptosis

Lid retraction

Pain on movement of extraocular muscles

Opthalmoplegia

Diplopia

Recent ocular malalignment

The red eye without obvious cause

Hyphema

Hypopyon

Abnormalities of the iris of recent onset

Irregularity of the iris

Abnormalities of the fundus

Corneal Abrasions

Corneal abrasions are another frequent cause of eye pain that prompts patients to seek urgent medical attention. The unique nature of the sensory innervation of the cornea results in the patient's perception of a foreign body in the eye any time the superficial corneal stroma is injured and the C-type polymodal nociceptors that richly innervate the cornea are stimulated. A foreign body sensation is usually felt by the

---

Box 4
Common causes of severe eye pain

Corneal ulcer

Uveitis

Acute angle closure glaucoma

Endophthalmitis

Scleritis

patient as being located under the upper eyelid even when no foreign body is present, and damage is limited to the corneal stroma. The continued firing of the polymodal receptors and recruitment of the corneal mechanoreceptors are probably responsible for this foreign body sensation, which occurs in almost all patients with corneal abrasion, even in the absence of a foreign body.

Patients with corneal abrasion usually relate a history of grit or a foreign body being blown into the eye or of minor mechanical trauma to the cornea during the insertion of contact lens or while playing sports.[7,8] Fluorescein staining usually reveals the damage to the corneal stroma; a foreign body is rarely seen.[9] The patient reports severe pain that is out of proportion to the apparent injury and insists that something is trapped under the upper eyelid, even after repeated attempts to convince the patient to the contrary. Photophobia and excessive lacrimation and scleral and conjunctival injection are often present, as is a significant substrate of anxiety.[6]

In the presence of corneal abrasion, the clinician should invert the upper eyelid and rinse the eye with copious amounts of sterile saline solution to remove any residual foreign body that may not be readily apparent on initial investigation. If the corneal abrasion is the result of an accident that occurred during hammering or the use of power tools, a careful search for a metallic foreign body should be undertaken and a plain radiograph or computed tomographic scan of the orbit and orbital contents should be obtained to rule out occult intraocular metallic foreign body, which can present a significant risk to vision if undetected. Treatment with non–neomycin-containing antibiotic ointment, such as gentamicin or polymyxin-B and bacitracin ophthalmic ointment, and a large dose of reassurance usually resolves the problem.[10] Most clinicians think that the disadvantages associated with the patching of the eye (eg, monocular vision, infection risk) outweigh the benefits in patients with small corneal abrasions.[11,12] Eye patching may be warranted in large, central corneal abrasions and consultation with a corneal specialist is advisable.[11]

Conjunctivitis

Infection of the conjunctiva is a common cause of eye pain. Caused by bacteria, fungus, or virus, conjunctivitis can range from a mild self-limited disease that requires no treatment to a purulent eye infection that can be quite uncomfortable and upsetting to the patient.[13] Bacterial and viral conjunctivitis, which is also known as pink eye, can be contagious, and all patients with conjunctivitis should be instructed in good hand-washing techniques and informed of the need to sterilize fomites that they have in common with the family and coworkers (eg, copy machines, faucets, telephones, computer keyboards). In addition to infectious causes, conjunctivitis can also be caused by environmental irritants, including pollen, dust, smog, and fumes.[14]

The patient with conjunctivitis presents with a red, irritated, and painful eye that is often associated with excessive lacrimation and some degree of photophobia.[6] A purulent discharge is also often present, especially if the cause is bacterial. If the discharge is severe, the patient may awaken with the eyelids stuck together, resulting in extreme anxiety for the patient and may result in a trip to the nearest emergency department for treatment. One factor that can help the clinician distinguish viral and bacterial cause is that preauricular adenopathy is a frequent finding in viral conjunctivitis but is almost never seen when a bacterial cause is present.[6] Treatment of acute conjunctivitis begins with reassurance and the use of a cold compresses to the affected eye to afford symptomatic relief.[6] If the cause is presumed bacterial, non–neomycin-containing antibiotic eye drops or ointment, such as polymyxin-B and bacitracin, or a fluoroquinolone (eg, moxifloxacin) should be used, with care being taken to avoid touching the affected eye with the dropper or the tip of the tube of antibiotic ointment to avoid reinfection.[15] If the patient wears contact lens, an antibiotic that covers pseudomonas, such as besifloxacin or levofloxacin, should be used. If the possibility of sexually transmitted conjunctivitis (eg, gonorrhea or chlamydia) is present, a culture should be taken, and appropriate systemic antibiotics and ophthalmologic consultation on an urgent basis are indicated because *Neisseria gonorrhea* can cause corneal destruction and tissue damage, which can be devastating to the eye.[16,17]

Episcleritis and Scleritis

Episcleritis and scleritis are common causes of eye pain; however, differentiating the 2 is of extreme importance as the latter can be devastating to vision if untreated.[18] Episcleritis is a self-limiting redness of the sclera that is acute in onset that does not involve pain or the pain is mild and dull in nature.[18] It is often recurrent and the cornea is not involved.[6] Frequently it is idiopathic and can be associated with collagen vascular diseases as well as herpes zoster and Lyme disease.[6] Scleritis, on the other hand, is a redness of the sclera that is characterized by severe pain that often radiates to the temple or jaw. It is often gradual in onset and the cornea can be affected.[6] It is often idiopathic but can be associated with autoimmune diseases and inflammatory conditions, such as rheumatoid arthritis, systemic lupus erythematosus, Wegener granulomatosis, and giant cell arteritis, and infections such as herpes zoster and Lyme disease.[18] Unlike episcleritis, scleritis is not self-limiting and can be destructive to the eye and to the patient's vision.[18] If either of these entities is suspected, immediate referral to the ophthalmologist is necessary for appropriate diagnosis and treatment, which typically involves systemic anti-inflammatory agents, such as nonsteroidal anti-inflammatory drugs or corticosteroids.[6]

Glaucoma

For purposes of this discussion, the clinician must be aware of the following 2 types of glaucoma: (1) open-angle glaucoma; and (2) angle-closure glaucoma.[19] A comparison of both types of this vision-threatening disease is provided in **Table 1**.

The clinician may encounter patients with eye pain and visual loss that may be the result of angle-closure glaucoma. Angle-closure glaucoma occurs when the angle between the iris and the cornea becomes blocked, impeding the drainage of aqueous humor (**Fig. 2**). Angle-closure glaucoma represents a true ophthalmologic emergency, and failure to identify the disease rapidly and to help the patient receive immediate ophthalmologic care invariably results in permanent visual loss.[20,21] The patient with acute angle-closure glaucoma presents with the acute onset of severe eye pain, blurred vision, a halo effect around lights, nausea and vomiting, and a red eye. The cornea may appear steamy, like looking though a steamy window. The pupil may be poorly reactive or fixed in mid position. The onset of angle-closure glaucoma frequently occurs at night or in dim light when the pupil dilates, further impeding the flow of the aqueous humor by further narrowing or closing the angle between the iris and the cornea.[18]

Management of acute angle closure is a medical emergency that requires immediate ophthalmologic referral for laser iridotomy and medical management with pressure-lowering agents.[6]

Uveitis

Uveitis is a term used to describe inflammation of the uveal tract from an infectious or noninfectious cause.[22] Uveitis is a common cause of eye pain, and the pain is frequently associated with a red eye and photophobia. Uveitis is frequently associated

Table 1
Comparison of open-angle and angle-closure glaucoma

	Open-Angle Glaucoma	Angle-Closure Glaucoma
Occurrence	85% of all glaucomas	15% of all glaucomas
Cause	Unknown	Closed angle prevents aqueous drainage
Age at onset	Variable	Age 50 y or older
Anterior chamber	Usually normal	Shallow
Chamber angle	Normal	Narrow
Symptoms	Insidious loss of vision, no pain early in disease	Acute pain, halos around lights, vomiting, headache
Cupping of disc	Progressive if untreated	After untreated attacks
Visual fields	Peripheral visual fields affected early, central vision affected later	Loss occurs as disease progresses
Ocular pressure	Progressively higher as disease progresses	High as disease progresses
Other signs	None	Fixed, partially dilated pupil, red eye, steamy cornea
Treatment	Medical, laser surgery	Surgical
Prognosis	Good if diagnosed early, poor if treatment delayed	Good if treated early, poor if treatment delayed

Modified from Swartz MH. Textbook of physical diagnosis. 4th edition. Philadelphia: Saunders; 2002. p. 235.

with autoimmune diseases (eg, rheumatoid arthritis, Behçet disease, human leukocyte antigen–positive anterior uveitis, Reiter syndrome, juvenile rheumatoid arthritis, inflammatory bowel disease), although the causes of uveitis may defy specific diagnosis (ie, idiopathic uveitis).[23] Infections, such as syphilis, toxoplasmosis, tuberculosis, Lyme disease, and human herpes virus, can also be to blame.[6] Other causes to consider are malignancies such as lymphoma and leukemia as well as trauma or

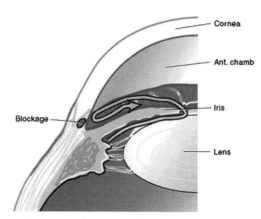

Fig. 2. Angle-closure glaucoma. (*From* Waldman SD. Pain management. 2nd edition. Elsevier; 2011. Figure 53-6.)

sarcoidosis.[6] Patients with uveitis present with eye pain, decreased vision, red eye, photophobia, blurred vision, and "floaters."[24] The pain of uveitis can be exacerbated by shining a bright light into the eye, causing the inflamed iris to constrict. Uveitis is an ophthalmologic emergency, and, if suspected, immediate ophthalmologic evaluation and treatment are mandatory if permanent visual loss is to be avoided.[25]

Endophthalmitis is a subclass of uveitis that involves inflammation of the vitreous, which is an important entity to recognize as it often involves severe eye pain and requires immediate ophthalmologic referral.[6] Endophthalmitis is frequently associated with recent eye surgery as well as trauma from a retained foreign body and less commonly infection from septic emboli or fungi.[6] Patients present with severe eye pain, decreased vision, and red eye. As noted, immediate ophthalmologic referral is needed as vision could be threatened.[6]

Optic Neuritis

Optic neuritis is another common cause of eye pain. Although pain is invariably present, it is the acute visual loss associated with the disease that usually prompts the patient to seek medical attention. The most common cause of optic neuritis is multiple sclerosis, with approximately 20% of patients with multiple sclerosis having optic neuritis as the initial symptom.[26] Approximately 70% of patients with multiple sclerosis have optic neuritis at some point in the disease.[27] Other causes of optic neuritis include temporal arteritis, tuberculosis, human immunodeficiency virus (HIV), hepatitis B, Lyme disease, and cytomegalovirus.[28] Optic neuritis is also seen with some medications, such as salycilates, digitalis, and amiodarone, and as a sequela to sinus infection (especially in children).[29] It can also occur after radiation therapy.[30]

Patients with optic neuritis present with a triad of symptoms, including the following: (1) acute vision loss; (2) eye pain, especially with eye movement; and (3) dyschromatopsia, which is an impairment of accurate color vision.[6] Some patients with optic neuritis also report sound-induced or sudden movement–induced flashing lights and heat-induced visual loss.[29] Approximately 70% of patients with optic neuritis have unilateral symptoms. On physical examination, the patient with optic neuritis exhibits a pale, swollen, optic disc as well as an afferent pupillary defect.[29,31–33] If the cause is believed to be due to multiple sclerosis, referral to neurology for treatment with intravenous methylprednisolone is indicated.[6] If the cause is believed to be infectious, then the appropriate antimicrobial therapy should be initiated.[29]

Refractive Errors

Patients often attribute their headache symptoms to eye strain, weak vision, and the like. Although refractive errors and eye strain are believed to cause headaches and are recognized causes by the International Headache Society, there is no definite evidence demonstrating a causal relationship.[52] Also, it can often be difficult to distinguish these causes from tension headaches or other headaches as both may coexist and are reasonably common.[34] In periods of intense eye use (eg, studying for finals, fine needlework, etc), the eye muscles begin to fatigue and the patient may begin to experience feelings of ocular and periocular discomfort, pressure, and eyelid heaviness.[34,52] Injection of the tarsal plates, conjunctival injection, and tearing is common. Low light situations may exacerbate the symptoms in some patients. If the patient continues to strain the eyes, a headache analogous to a tension-type headache can occur.[34] In children, headaches are often attributed to eye strain, and, although an association between the 2 has been recognized, it is rare, thus leading to an overdiagnosis of this condition.[6,52]

REFERRED EYE PAIN
Cluster Headache

Cluster headache is a common cause of referred ocular and periocular pain. The presumption is that interplay between the sphenopalatine ganglion and the trigeminal ganglion is responsible for the patient's perception of eye pain with cluster headache. Cluster headache derives its name from the pattern of its occurrence: namely, the headaches occur in clusters followed by headache-free remission periods.[35] Unlike other common headache disorders that affect primarily women, cluster headache occurs much more often in men, by a ratio of 5:1. Much less common than tension-type headache or migraine headache, cluster headache is thought to affect approximately 0.5% of the male population.

The onset of cluster headache occurs in the late third or early fourth decade, in contradistinction to migraine, which almost always manifests by the early second decade. Unlike migraine, cluster headache does not seem to run in families, and cluster headache sufferers do not experience aura. Attacks of cluster headache generally occur approximately 90 minutes after the patient falls asleep. This association with sleep is reportedly maintained when a shift worker changes to and from nighttime to daytime hours of sleep. Cluster headache also seems to follow a distinct chronobiologic pattern that coincides with the seasonal change in the length of daylight, resulting in an increased frequency of cluster headaches in the spring and fall.

During a cluster headache period, attacks occur 2 to 3 times a day and last for 45 minutes to an hour. Cluster headache periods usually last for 8 to 12 weeks, interrupted by remission periods of less than 2 years. In rare cases, the remission periods become shorter and shorter and the frequency may increase up to 10-fold. This situation is termed chronic cluster headache and differs from the more common episodic cluster headache described previously.

Cluster headache is characterized as a unilateral headache that is ocular, retroorbital, and temporal. The pain has a deep burning or boring quality. Physical findings during an attack of cluster headache may include Horner syndrome, consisting of ptosis, abnormal pupil constriction, facial flushing, and conjunctival injection. In addition, profuse lacrimation and rhinorrhea are often present. The ocular changes may become permanent with repeated attacks. Peau d'orange skin over the malar region, deeply furrowed and glabellar folds, and telangiectasia may be observed.

Attacks of cluster headache may be provoked by small amounts of alcohol, nitrates, histamines, and other vasoactive substances and occasionally by high altitude. When the attack is in progress, the patient may not be able to lie still and may pace or rock back and forth in a chair. This behavior contrasts to that in other headache syndromes, during which patients seeking relief lie down in a dark quiet room.

The pain of cluster headache is said to be among the worst pain that mankind suffers. Because of the severity of pain associated with cluster headaches, the clinician must watch closely for medication overuse or misuse. Suicides have been associated with prolonged, unrelieved attacks of cluster headaches.

No specific test for cluster headache exists. Testing is aimed primarily at identifying occult pathologic abnormalities or other diseases that may mimic cluster headache. All patients with a recent onset of headache thought to be cluster headache should undergo magnetic resonance imaging (MRI) testing of the brain. Screening laboratory testing, including erythrocyte sedimentation rate, complete blood cell count, and automated blood chemistry, should be performed if the diagnosis of cluster headache is in question. Ophthalmologic evaluation including measurement of intraocular pressures is indicated in those patients with headache who experience significant ocular symptoms.

In contradistinction to migraine headache, where most patients experience improvement with the implementation of therapy with β-adrenergic blockers, patients with cluster headache usually need more individualized therapy. A reasonable starting place in the treatment of cluster headache is to begin treatment with prednisone combined with daily sphenopalatine ganglion blocks with local anesthetic.[36] A reasonable starting dose of prednisone is 80 mg given in divided doses tapered by 10 mg per dose per day. If headaches are not rapidly brought under control, the inhalation of 100% oxygen is added via a close-fitting mask.

If headaches persist and the diagnosis of cluster headache is not in question, a trial of lithium carbonate may be considered. Note that the therapeutic window of lithium carbonate is small and thus this drug should be used with caution. A starting dose of 300 mg at bedtime may be increased after 48 hours to 300 mg twice a day. If no side effects are noted after 48 hours, the dose may again be increased to 300 mg 3 times a day. The patient should be continued at this dosage level for a total of 10 days, and the drug should then be tapered downward over a 1-week period. Other medications that can be considered if the aforementioned treatments are ineffective include methysergide, sumatriptan, and sumatriptan-like drugs.

Tolosa-Hunt Syndrome

Tolosa-Hunt syndrome is another disease with a primary presenting symptom of unilateral eye pain. The exact cause of Tolosa-Hunt syndrome is unknown, but the ocular and periocular symptoms are the result of nonspecific inflammation of the cavernous sinus or superior orbital fissure.[37] In addition to severe eye pain, which often heralds the onset of this disease, dysfunction of cranial nerves III, IV, and VI occurs as a result of granulomatous inflammatory damage to the nerves,[38] resulting in ophthalmoparesis, which can be quite distressing to the patient. In some patients, the ophthalmoparesis may precede the pain, further confusing the diagnosis. Pupillary dysfunction from inflammation of the sympathetic fibers and third cranial nerve may also be seen in patients with Tolosa-Hunt syndrome. If the inflammation extends beyond the cavernous sinus and affects the optic nerve, blindness may result. Paresthesias into the forehead presumably via the supraorbital branch of the trigeminal nerve may also be present as part of the inflammatory response. Tolosa-Hunt syndrome rarely occurs before the second decade and affects men and women equally. The extent of physical findings is a direct function of which cranial nerves are affected by the inflammatory process. Although ophthalmopareses is a hallmark of Tolosa-Hunt syndrome, papillary abnormalities and ptosis may also be present. Fundoscopic examination may reveal edema of the optic disc.[39] The corneal reflex may be diminished or lost if significant trigeminal nerve involvement occurs.

Because Tolosa-Hunt syndrome mimics many other diseases, laboratory testing, including a complete blood cell count and determination of erythrocyte sedimentation rate, glucose level, Lyme disease titer, rapid plasma reagin, antinuclear antibody, HIV titer, and thyroid function, is indicated.[40] MRI of the brain and orbit may reveal findings suggestive of a local inflammatory response but may be normal even in the presence of significant disease.[41] Biopsy of the region of inflammation may ultimately be necessary to confirm the diagnosis of Tolosa-Hunt syndrome. Tolosa-Hunt syndrome represents an ophthalmologic emergency and should be treated as such. Rapid treatment with high doses of intravenous corticosteroids may prevent loss of vision and cranial nerve function. Although spontaneous remissions have been reported, early treatment is key to avoiding disastrous results. Thirty percent to 40% of patients with Tolosa-Hunt syndrome experience a relapse of symptoms after successful treatment with corticosteroids.

The Cavernous Sinus Syndromes

The cavernous sinus syndromes are a heterogeneous group of diseases that have in common their ability to produce ocular and periocular pain and a variety of neurologic symptoms, including ophthalmoplegia, pupillary abnormalities, orbital and conjunctival congestion, proptosis, and, if severe, visual loss.[42] Also known as the parasellar syndromes, the evaluation of all patients with cavernous sinus syndrome should include a complete blood cell count and determination of erythrocyte sedimentation rate, glucose level, Lyme disease titer, rapid plasma reagin, antinuclear antibody, HIV titer, and thyroid function. MRI of the brain, sinuses, cavernous sinus, and orbit is also indicated as is magnetic resonance angiography of the carotid artery. Diseases that comprise the cavernous sinus syndrome include cavernous sinus aneurysms, carotid-cavernous sinus fistulas, tumors, and cavernous sinus thrombosis, and the idiopathic inflammatory syndromes that involve the cavernous sinus (eg, Tolosa-Hunt syndrome).[43,44]

Cavernous Sinus Aneurysms

Aneurysms of the carotid artery as it passes through the cavernous sinus can cause all of the symptoms associated with cavernous sinus syndrome. Unlike intracranial aneurysms, which carry the risk of intracranial hemorrhage, unruptured carotid artery aneurysms in this region create symptoms with pressure on the various neural structures in proximity to the aneurysm. When the aneurysm ruptures, a direct carotid artery–cavernous sinus fistula results. Such fistulas can cause only limited symptoms or can result in massive neurologic dysfunction. A loud carotid and ocular bruit is often present. Treatment with endovascular occlusion has been attempted with some success.[45]

Cavernous Sinus Tumors

Tumors that involve the cavernous sinus can be either primary or metastatic in origin. Primary tumors including meningiomas and neurofibromas are the most common primary tumors seen that involve the cavernous sinus.[46,47] Occasionally, large pituitary tumors may extend into the cavernous sinus. Symptoms associated with tumors of this region vary with the neurologic structures affected as the tumor grows, and the onset of symptoms can be either acute or insidious. Treatment is primarily limited to palliative radiotherapy, and the results in most cases are poor at best, with the type of tumor the major determinant of outcome. The exception to this rule is endocrine-responsive pituitary tumors, which often respond to antiendocrine drug therapy.

Carotid-Cavernous Fistulas

Direct fistulas between the carotid artery and the cavernous sinus occur when a carotid artery aneurysm ruptures directly into the cavernous sinus or trauma to the region damages the artery.[48] The onset of symptoms is immediate and often quite severe. Misdiagnosis is common, and prognosis if untreated is poor. A loud carotid and ocular bruit is often present. The patient may report hearing "water running" in the head. Indirect aneurysms between branches of the internal or external carotid arteries tend to be less symptomatic. Both types of fistulas can be treated with endovascular occlusion techniques and carotid artery ligation.

Cavernous Sinus Thrombosis

A common sequela to periorbital or frontal or maxillary sinusitis in the preantibiotic era, cavernous sinus thrombosis is now primarily seen in immunocompromised patients (eg, patients with HIV).[49] The patient with an infectious cause to cavernous sinus thrombosis appears septic, and the nidus of the infection may be clinically evident. Severe ocular and retroocular pain is often the first symptom, followed by diplopia and ptosis. Ophthalmoplegia and signs of meningeal irritation may also be present. Immediate treatment with antibiotics and corticosteroids combined with surgical drainage of any abscess formation is crucial to avoid blindness or, in some cases, death.

Other Inflammatory Conditions Associated with Cavernous Sinus Syndrome

Acute herpes zoster and sarcoidosis have both been implicated in the development of cavernous sinus syndrome. The lesions of acute herpes zoster usually make the diagnosis a relatively straightforward endeavor, but the diagnosis of sarcoidosis can be much more subtle.[50,51] If uveitis is present as a component of ocular pain, sarcoidosis should always be included in the differential diagnosis.

REFERENCES

1. Waldman SD. Gasserian ganglion block. In: Waldman SD, editor. Atlas of interventional pain management. 3rd edition. Philadelphia: Saunders; 2009. p. 32–3.
2. Muller LJ. Corneal nerves: structure, contents, and function. Exp Eye Res 2003; 76:521.
3. Pavan-Langston D. Diagnosis and therapy of common eye infections: bacterial, viral, fungal. Compr Ther 1983;9:33.
4. Barza M, Baum J. Ocular infections. Med Clin North Am 1983;407:131.
5. Briner AM. Surgical treatment of a chalazion or hordeolum internum. Aust Fam Physician 1987;16:834.
6. Palay DA, Krachmer J. Primary care ophthalmology. 2nd edition. Philadelphia: Elsevier; 2005.
7. Burke MJ, Sanitato JJ, Vinger PF, et al. Soccerball-induced eye injuries. JAMA 1983;213:2682.
8. Stapleton F, Dart J, Minassian D. Nonulcerative complications of contact lens wear: relative risks for different lens types. Arch Ophthalmol 1992;110:1601.
9. Brunette DD, Ghezzi K, Benner GS. Ophthalmologic disorders. In: Rosen P, Barkin R, editors. Emergency medicine: concepts and clinical practice. 4th edition. St Louis (MO): Mosby; 1997. p. 2432–40.
10. Patterson J, Fetzer D, Krall J, et al. Eye patch treatment for the pain of corneal abrasion. South Med J 1996;89:227.
11. Turner A, Rabiu M. Patching for corneal abrasion. Cochrane Database Syst Rev 2006;(2):CD004764. http://dx.doi.org/10.1002/14651858.CD004764.pub2.
12. Spiegel D. Primary open-angle glaucoma. In: Dartt DA, editor. Encyclopedia of the eye. Oxford (United Kingdom): Academic Press; 2010. p. 496–501.
13. Bertolini J, Pelucio M. The red eye. Emerg Med Clin North Am 1995;13:561.
14. Friedlaender MH. The current and future therapy of allergic conjunctivitis. Curr Opin Ophthalmol 1998;9:54.
15. Steinert RF. Current therapy for bacterial keratitis and bacterial conjunctivitis. Am J Ophthalmol 1991;112(Suppl 4):10S–4S.
16. Bersudsky V, Rehany U, Tendler Y. Diagnosis of chlamydial infection by direct enzyme-linked immunoassay and polymerase chain reaction in patients with acute follicular conjunctivitis. Graefes Arch Clin Exp Ophthalmol 1999;237:617.

17. Salmon JF. Glaucoma. In: Riordan-Eva P, Witcher JP, editors. General ophthalmology. 17th edition. New York: McGraw-Hill; 2008. p. 212–28.
18. Spalton DJ. Atlas of Clinical Ophthalmology. 3rd edition. Philadelphia: Vendome; 2005.
19. Mitchell JD. Ocular emergencies. In: Tintinalli, editor. Emergency medicine: a comprehensive study guide. 5th edition. New York: McGraw-Hill; 2000. p. 1501–17.
20. Choong YF, Irfan S, Menage MJ. Acute angle closure glaucoma: an evaluation of a protocol for acute treatment. Eye 1999;13:613.
21. Campbell DG. A comparison of diagnostic techniques in angle-closure glaucoma. Am J Ophthalmol 1979;88:197.
22. Nussenblatt R, Whitcup S, Palestine A. Uveitis: fundamentals of clinical practice. 2nd edition. St Louis (MO): Mosby; 1996.
23. Pepose JS, Holland GN, Wilhelmus KR. Ocular infection and immunity. St Louis (MO): Mosby; 1996.
24. Tessler H. Classification and symptoms and signs of uveitis. In: Duane T, editor. Clinical ophthalmology. New York: Harper & Row; 1987. p. 1–10.
25. Nishimoto JY. Iritis: how to recognize and manage a potentially sight-threatening disease. Postgrad Med 1996;99:255.
26. Kidd DP, Plant GT. Optic neuritis. Blue Books Neurol 2008;32:134–52.
27. Noseworthy JH, Lucchinetti C, Rodriguez M, et al. Multiple sclerosis. N Engl J Med 2000;343:938.
28. Ghezzi A, Martinelli V, Rodegher M, et al. The prognosis of idiopathic optic neuritis. Neurol Sci 2000;21(4 Suppl 2):S865.
29. Dartt DA. Encyclopedia of the eye. New York: Elsevier; 2010. p. 205–9.
30. Danesh-Meyer HV. Radiation-induced optic neuropathy. J Clin Neurosci 2008; 15(2):95–100.
31. Miller DH, Newton MR, van der Poel JC, et al. Magnetic resonance imaging of the optic nerve in optic neuritis. Neurology 1988;38:175.
32. Biousse V, Calvetti O, Drews-Botsch CD, et al. Management of optic neuritis and impact of clinical trials: an international survey. J Neurol Sci 2009;276(1–2): 69–74.
33. Jacobs LD, Beck RW, Simon JH, et al. Intramuscular interferon beta-1a therapy initiated during a first demyelinating event in multiple sclerosis: CHAMPS Study Group. N Engl J Med 2000;343:898.
34. Akinci A, Güven A, Degerliyurt A. The correlation between headache and refractive errors. J AAPOS 2008;12(3):290–3.
35. Waldman SD. Cluster headache. In: Waldman SD, editor. Common pain syndromes. 2nd edition. Philadelphia: Saunders; 2008. p. 14–6.
36. Waldman SD. Sphenopalatine ganglion block. In: Waldman SD, editor. Atlas of interventional pain management. 3rd edition. Philadelphia: Saunders; 2009. p. 12–4.
37. Cohn DF, Carasso R, Streifler M. Painful ophthalmoplegia: the Tolosa-Hunt syndrome. Eur Neurol 1979;18:373.
38. Roca PD. Painful ophthalmoplegia: the Tolosa-Hunt syndrome. Ann Ophthalmol 1975;7:828.
39. Hunt WE. Tolosa-Hunt syndrome: one cause of painful ophthalmoplegia. J Neurosurg 1976;44:544.
40. Troost BT. Comprehensive and infiltrative optic neuropathies. In: Miller NR, Newman NJ, editors. Walsh & Hoyt's clinical neuro-ophthalmology. Philadelphia: Lippincott Williams & Wilkins; 1998. p. 1727–9.
41. Yousem DM, Atlas SW, Grossman RI. MR imaging of Tolosa-Hunt syndrome. AJR Am J Roentgenol 1990;154:167.

42. Thomas JE, Yoss RE. The parasellar syndrome: problems in determining etiology. Mayo Clin Proc 1970;45:617.
43. Hunt WE, Meagher JN, Lefever HE, et al. Painful ophthalmoplegia: its relation to indolent inflammation of the cavernous sinus. Neurology 1961;11:56.
44. Kline LB. The Tolosa-Hunt syndrome. Surv Ophthalmol 1982;119:79.
45. Kupersmith MJ, Berenstein A, Choi IS, et al. Percutaneous transvascular treatment of giant carotid aneurysms: neuro-ophthalmologic findings. Neurology 1984;34:328.
46. Kattah JC, Silgals RM, Manz H, et al. Presentation and management of parasellar and suprasellar metastatic mass lesions. J Neurol Neurosurg Psychiatry 1985;48:44.
47. Greenberg HS, Deck MD, Vikram B, et al. Metastasis to the base of the skull: clinical findings in 43 patients. Neurology 1981;31:130.
48. Debrun G, Lacour P, Vinuela F, et al. Treatment of 54 traumatic carotid-cavernous fistulas. J Neurosurg 1981;55:678.
49. Hedges TR, Leung LS. Parasellar and orbital apex syndrome caused by aspergillosis. Neurology 1976;26:117.
50. Belfer MH, Stevens RW. Sarcoidosis: a primary care review. Am Fam Physician 1998;58:2041.
51. Buttaravoli P. Hordeolum. Minor Emergencies 2007;19:85–6.

Headache Pain of Ear, Nose, Throat, and Sinus Origin

Steven D. Waldman, MD, JD[a],*, Corey W. Waldman, MD[b],
Jennifer E. Waldman[c]

KEYWORDS

- Mastoiditis • Otitis externa • Maxillary sinusitis • Tension type headache
- Eagle syndrome

KEY POINTS

- Infection should be a primary concern in all patients suffering from headache pain attributed to the ear, nose, and throat.
- More often than not, the patient's headache symptomatology can be attributed to a primary headache cause such as tension-type headache.
- Sinus headache is grossly overdiagnosed and treated.
- Familiarity with less common abnormalities of the ear, nose, and throat will often simplify the diagnosis of the patient's headache pain.

Pain that originates in the ear, nose, sinuses, and throat accounts for a significant number of visits each year to primary care physicians and specialists. Often these painful conditions are described by the patient as headache, and if not severe tend to be initially self-treated with over-the-counter remedies. Although most of the painful conditions responsible for these visits are easy to diagnose and treat and, in general, will not harm the patient with proper treatment, a significant number of painful conditions of the ear, nose, and throat have the potential to cause considerable morbidity and mortality (**Box 1**). The clinician should also remain vigilant for diseases of this anatomic region that do not cause pain but have the potential, if undiagnosed, to create significant problems for the patient, such as acoustic neuroma, thyroid carcinoma, and malignant melanoma. This article provides the clinician with a concise road map for the evaluation of painful conditions of the ear, nose, sinuses, and throat that may be responsible for headache.

Large portions of this text were originally published in Waldman SD. Pain of the Ear, Nose, Sinus and Throat. In: Waldman SD, editor. Pain Management. 2nd Edition. Chapter 54: Elsevier; 2011. p. 494–502.

[a] School of Medicine, University of Missouri-Kansas City, 2411 Holmes, Kansas City, Missouri, MO 64108, USA; [b] Krieger Eye Institute At Sinai, 2411 West Belvedere Avenue, Baltimore, USA; [c] Brain Tissue Bank, School of Medicine, University of Missouri-Kansas City, Kansas City, Missouri, USA
* Corresponding author.
E-mail address: sdwaldmanmd@gmail.com

Med Clin N Am 97 (2013) 309–319
http://dx.doi.org/10.1016/j.mcna.2012.12.005
0025-7125/13/$ – see front matter © 2013 Elsevier Inc. All rights reserved.

Box 1
Painful conditions of the ear, nose, sinuses, and throat

EAR PAIN

    The Auricle

        Superficial infections

        Folliculitis

        Cellulitis

        Herpes simplex

        Ramsay Hunt syndrome

        Deep infections involving cartilage

        Trauma

        Ecchymosis of the auricle

        Perichondral hematoma

        Lacerations

        Thermal injuries

        Heating-pad burns

        Ice-pack burns

        Frostbite

        Chondritis-associated and perichondritis-associated connective tissue diseases

        Primary tumors

        Metastatic tumors

    The External Auditory Canal

        Otitis media

        Cholesteatoma

    The Tympanic Membrane and Middle Ear

        Myringitis

        Otitis media

        Mastoiditis

PAIN OF THE NOSE AND SINUSES

    Superficial infection

    Folliculitis

    Vestibulitis

    Intranasal foreign body

    Acute sinusitis

    Osteomyelitis

    Primary tumors of the nose and sinuses

    Metastatic tumors involving the nose and sinuses

THROAT PAIN

    Superficial infection

    Acute pharyngitis

Tonsillitis

Dental pain

Deep infection

Parapharyngeal abscess

Retropharyngeal abscess

Primary tumors of the throat and aerodigestive tract

Metastatic tumors involving the throat and aerodigestive tract

Carotidynia

Eagle syndrome

Hyoid syndrome

From Waldman SD. Pain management. 2nd edition. Elsevier: 2011. Table 54-1.

OTALGIA

Ear pain can result from local abnormality, such as cellulitis or tumor, or can be referred from distant sites, most commonly the nasopharynx.[1,2] Because of the complex functions of the ear, local disease may cause disturbances in hearing and balance that can be distressing for the patient and may serve as a harbinger of serious diseases, such as acoustic neuroma. As mentioned, many of these conditions do not have pain as a predominant symptom.

Functional Anatomy of the Ear as it Relates to Pain

The ear and surrounding tissues are innervated by both cranial nerves and branches of nerves that have as their origin the spinal nerves (**Fig. 1**). The auricle is innervated by the greater auricular nerve and the lesser occipital nerve, the auricular branch of the vagus nerve, and the auriculotemporal branch of the mandibular nerve. The external auditory canal receives innervation from branches of the glossopharyngeal and facial nerves. The inferoposterior portion of the tympanic membrane receives its innervation from the auriculotemporal branch of the mandibular nerve, the auricular branch of the vagus nerve, and the tympanic branch of the glossopharyngeal nerve. The structures of the middle ear receive innervation from the tympanic branch of the glossopharyngeal nerve along with the caroticotympanic nerve and the superficial petrosal nerve. It is the overlap of these nerves, and their diverse origin, that can make challenging the localization of the abnormality responsible for the patient's pain.

Painful Diseases of the Ear

Auricular pain

The skin of the auricle is richly innervated and is frequently the source of local ear pain. Auricular cartilage is poorly innervated, and diseases that are limited to cartilage may produce little or no pain until distention or inflammation of the overlying skin develops. Most painful conditions involving the auricle are the result of infection, trauma, connective tissue disease, or tumor.

Superficial infections of the auricle include folliculitis, abscess, cellulitis, and infection by herpes simplex and zoster, including Ramsay Hunt syndrome.[3] Deep infections that involve the cartilage, once uncommon, now occur with much greater frequency because of the current increase in body piercing involving auricular cartilage.

Both superficial and deep infections of the auricle are painful. Early incision and drainage, débridement of nonviable cartilage, and aggressive use of antibiotics are

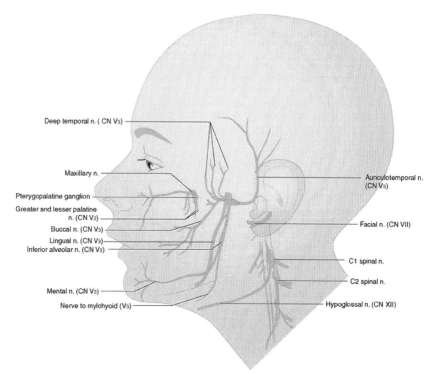

Fig. 1. Innervation of the ear and surrounding tissues. (*From* Waldman SD. Pain management. 2nd edition. Elsevier: 2011. Figure 54-1.)

necessary to avoid spread of infection to the middle ear, bone, and intracranial structures, including the central nervous system.

Trauma to the auricle can be painful and, if not appropriately treated, can result in loss of cartilage and disfigurement. Blunt trauma to the auricle can cause superficial ecchymosis or, if severe enough, perichondral hematoma or cauliflower ear (**Fig. 2**).[4] Lacerations of the lobule, tragus, and cartilage from body piercings that

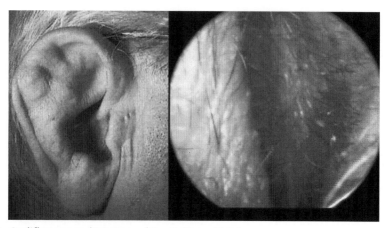

Fig. 2. Cauliflower ear. (*Courtesy of* Roy Sullivan, PhD.)

have been torn from the ear are increasingly common occurrences at local emergency rooms and urgent care centers. Prompt débridement and repair with careful observation for infection are crucial if disfiguring sequelae are to be avoided.

Thermal injuries from heat or cold are also common painful traumatic injuries to the ear that usually follow the use of heating pads or cold packs in patients who are also taking pain medications or self-medicating with alcohol, or both. Frostbite injuries that affect the auricle are likewise common, and are frequently related to alcohol or drug use (or both). Thermal injuries can initially appear less severe than they really are. Initial treatment with topical antibiotics such as silver sulfadiazine and sterile dressings should be followed with reevaluation and redressing of the affected area on a daily basis until the thermal injury is well on the way to healing.

Connective tissue diseases can cause inflammation of the auricular cartilage. Usually manifesting as bilateral, acutely inflamed, and painful swelling of the auricle, chondritis and perichondritis may initially be misdiagnosed as cellulitis (**Fig. 3**). The bilateral nature of the disease and the involvement of other cartilage should alert the clinician to the possibility of a noninfectious cause of the pain, rubor, and swelling.[5] Because many of the connective tissue diseases affect other organ systems, prompt diagnosis and treatment are essential.

Primary tumors of the auricle are generally basal cell or squamous cell carcinoma caused by actinic damage to the skin (**Fig. 4**). Rarely, primary tumors of the cartilage can occur. Metastatic lesions to the auricle are uncommon, but not unheard of.

The external auditory canal

By far the most common painful condition of the external auditory meatus is otitis externa. Usually the result of swimming or digging in the ear with a fingernail, cotton swab, or hairpin, the initial symptom of otitis media is generally pruritus, followed by pain that is made worse by yawning or chewing. On physical examination a reddened,

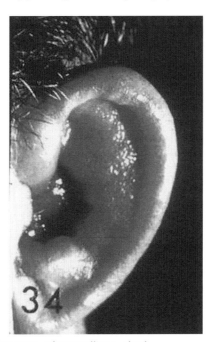

Fig. 3. Polychondritis. (*Courtesy of* Roy Sullivan, PhD.)

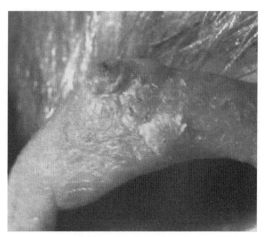

Fig. 4. Basal cell carcinoma. (*Courtesy of* Roy Sullivan, PhD.)

wet-appearing, edematous canal may reveal abraded areas from previous digging or itching as a result of the patient's attempt to relieve the symptoms (**Fig. 5**).[6] Pulling on the auricle posteriorly usually exacerbates the pain of otitis media. The pain of this disease is often disproportionate to the findings on physical examination. Treatment of otitis media consists of cleaning any debris from the acoustic auditory canal and instilling topical antibiotic drops or solution. If significant edema is present, the use of topical antibiotic drops or solution containing corticosteroid speeds recovery.

Another cause of external auditory canal pain is cholesteatoma, which most often occurs after trauma to the bone of the external auditory canal. Caused by invasion of the external auditory canal wall by exuberant tissue growth, cholesteatoma can become invasive if left untreated, despite its benign tissue elements.[7] A patient with cholesteatoma has a ball-like growth in the external auditory canal that has an onion-skin–like appearance (**Fig. 6**). Unless infected, the pain most often is dull and aching. Secondary infection may cause a foul-smelling purulent exudate to drain from the affected ear. Computed tomography (CT) helps the clinician determine the

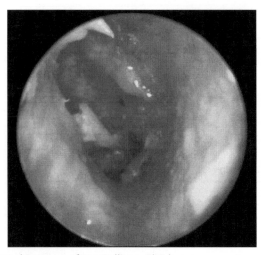

Fig. 5. Otitis externa. (*Courtesy of* Roy Sullivan, PhD.)

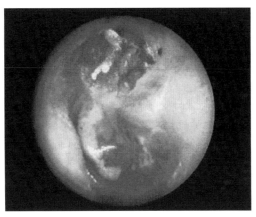

Fig. 6. Cholesteatoma. (*Courtesy of* Roy Sullivan, PhD.)

amount of bone destruction and helps guide microsurgical resection of this not uncommon cause of ear pain.

In younger patients and those with impaired mentation, foreign bodies are a frequently overlooked cause of ear pain originating from the external auditory meatus. Most problematic is vegetable matter, such as dried peas and beans, which swells once inside the acoustic auditory canal and makes removal difficult. If the foreign body remains in the external auditory canal for any period, secondary infection invariably occurs. Insects may also fly or crawl into the external auditory meatus and cause the patient much distress (**Fig. 7**). If the insect remains alive, instillation of lidocaine or mineral oil stops the insect from moving around and makes removal easier.[8]

The tympanic membrane and middle ear

Myringitis is a painful condition that may be caused by viral infection of the tympanic membrane. Vesicles or blebs of the tympanic membrane may be present on physical examination, or the tympanic membrane may appear normal. Antibiotic drops containing local anesthetic usually provide symptomatic relief, although in the absence

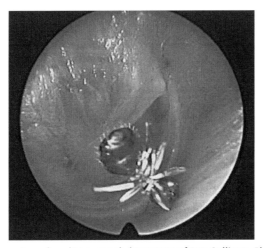

Fig. 7. Insect in the external auditory canal. (*Courtesy of* Roy Sullivan, PhD.)

of physical findings the diagnosis of idiopathic myringitis is one of exclusion, and other diseases of the middle ear or referred pain remain an ever-present possibility.

Acute otitis media is perhaps the second most common cause of otalgia after otitis externa. Although more common in children, otitis media can occur at any age. The pain of otitis media is caused primarily by distention and inflammation of the tympanic membrane **(Fig. 8)**.[9] Young children with otitis media may pull on the ear, whereas older patients report a deep, severe, unremitting pain. Fever is also usually present. Untreated, the pain becomes increasingly severe as the tympanic membrane becomes more distended until the tympanic membrane ruptures. Although the pain may dramatically improve after spontaneous rupture, infection of the mastoid air cells can occur. Treatment of acute otitis media is based on the administration of oral antibiotics and decongestants. Topical local anesthetic drops administered via the external auditory canal may provide symptomatic relief while waiting for the antibiotics and decongestants to work. For otitis media that does not promptly resolve, therapeutic tympanocentesis with the placement of myringotomy tubes should be considered.

As mentioned previously, acute mastoiditis is often the result of untreated or undertreated otitis media. Mastoiditis is characterized by pain, tenderness, and rubor in the posterior auricular region.[10] The condition is often misdiagnosed initially as recurrent otitis media because examination of the tympanic membrane often reveals findings of the unresolved otitis media. Fever is invariably present, and the patient generally appears more ill than with otitis media alone. Radiographic examination of the mastoid air cells reveals opacification of the normally aerated structure and, as the disease progresses, bony destruction. Untreated, mastoiditis can become life threatening as the infection spreads to the central nervous system (CNS). The findings of headache, stiff neck, and visual disturbance are warning signs of CNS involvement and constitute a medical emergency. Surgical treatment combined with aggressive antibiotic therapy is necessary on an emergency basis for patients with signs of CNS infection.

A word of caution is in order whenever the clinician is unable to identify the cause of a patient's ear pain. Idiopathic otalgia, especially if unilateral, is a diagnosis of exclusion that should generally be resisted because it is invariably wrong.[11] Repeat physical examination and careful retaking of the history, with special attention directed to areas

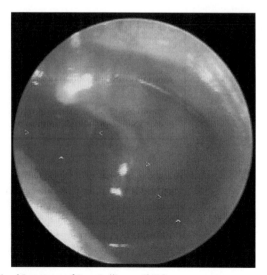

Fig. 8. Otitis media. (*Courtesy of* Roy Sullivan, PhD.)

where occult tumor might cause pain that is referred to the ear, are essential if disaster is to be avoided. This clinical situation is one whereby serial magnetic resonance imaging (MRI) of the brain and soft tissues of the neck, and CT scan of these areas, often yields results. All patients with unexplained ear pain should undergo careful endoscopic examination of the aerodigestive tract, with special attention paid to the region of the piriform sinuses to identify any occult abnormality that may be responsible for the pain (see later discussion).

PAIN OF THE NOSE AND SINUSES

Infection of the nose is the most common cause of nasal pain in the absence of trauma. Superficial soft-tissue infections can be painful and have the potential to spread to deep structures if left untreated. Folliculitis of the vestibule of the nose can also be very painful and, when caused by *Staphylococcus*, can be difficult to treat.[12–14] This condition has been occurring more commonly as the use of intranasal steroid sprays to treat atrophic rhinitis increases, and the early use of topical intranasal antibiotics, such as mupirocin, at the first sign of intranasal tenderness can help prevent more severe disease. Persistent foul-smelling discharge from the nose should alert the physician to the possibility of an intranasal foreign body, especially in children or mentally impaired individuals.

Acute sinusitis is another painful condition of the mid face that can be caused by all infectious agents. Blockage of the ostia of the sinus is usually the cause of acute sinusitis, with pressure within the sinuses increasing because mucus from the affected sinuses cannot flow into the nose. The maxillary sinuses are most commonly affected, and the pain associated with this disease can be severe. The pain is usually localized to the area over the sinus and may be worse with recumbency.

Treatment with decongestant nasal sprays and antibiotics resolves most cases of acute sinusitis. Untreated, osteomyelitis may occur. Surgery may ultimately be necessary for recurrent disease, for disease that remains unresponsive to conservative therapy, or when radiographs reveal obstructive polyps or tumors.

Malignant diseases of the nose and sinuses can be notoriously difficult to diagnose. The most common tumors of the nose are basal cell and squamous cell carcinoma.[15] Usually not painful unless infection intervenes or a painful structure is invaded, these tumors can become quite large before detection. Squamous cell carcinoma of the sinuses is manifested in a manner identical to sinusitis, so the diagnosis is often delayed. Nasopharyngoma occurs most commonly in patients of Asian descent. Thought to be caused by Epstein-Barr virus, these tumors frequently cause referred pain to the face, neck, and retroauricular area. Other lesions known for their ability to cause referred nose and facial pain are tumors that involve the parapharyngeal space.[16] Almost always causing unilateral symptoms such as facial paralysis and pain, parapharyngeal tumors are frequently of neural origin. As previously mentioned, delay in the diagnosis of these tumors can complicate treatment and worsen the prognosis.

THROAT PAIN

Pain that emanates from this region is poorly localized because of mixed innervation of the anatomic structures by the trigeminal, glossopharyngeal, and vagus nerves, and rich innervation by the sympathetic nervous system. For this reason, referred pain from this region is not the exception but the rule. Because of the patient's difficulty in accurately localizing the source of the pain when this anatomic region is affected, extra vigilance on the part of the clinician is needed.

Both superficial and deep infections are a common source of throat pain. Acute pharyngitis and laryngotracheobronchitis are among the most common reasons why patients seek medical attention.[17] Dental infections are also common causes of pain in this anatomic region, and often cause pain referred to the ear.[18] Generally self-limited, these infections can become problematic if they spread to the deep structures of the neck and aerodigestive tract or if they occur in immunocompromised patients. In particular, abscesses of the parapharyngeal and retropharyngeal space after acute pharyngitis and tonsillitis can become life threatening if not promptly diagnosed and treated.[19] Patients with these disorders appear acutely ill and talk with a characteristic muffled "hot-potato voice." With the increased availability of MRI and CT, early diagnosis of parapharyngeal and retropharyngeal abscesses is much easier.

In addition to infections, tumors of this region can produce both local and referred pain.[20] These tumors are often hard to diagnose, and by the time the pain is so severe that it causes the patient to seek medical attention, the tumors are already extremely problematic and in many cases have already metastasized. Most primary tumors in this region are squamous cell tumors, although primary tumors of the neural structures and craniopharyngiomas occur with sufficient frequency to be part of the differential diagnosis. Metastatic lesions can also cause local and referred pain in this anatomic area. Given the silent nature of this area insofar as symptoms are concerned, the clinician should make early and frequent use of MRI and CT to identify occult tumors and other pathologic factors.[21] In particular, the clinician should never attribute pain in this region to an idiopathic or psychogenic cause without serial physical examinations, laboratory evaluations, and imaging. In particular, unilateral otalgia in the absence of demonstrable ear abnormality should be taken seriously, and considered to be referred pain from occult tumor until proved otherwise.

Other painful conditions unrelated to infection and tumor can also occur in this anatomic region, including Eagle syndrome, carotidynia, and hyoid syndrome.

Eagle syndrome is caused by calcification of the stylohyoid ligament, and is characterized by paroxysms of pain with movement of the mandible during chewing, yawning, and talking.[22] Carotidynia consists of deep neck pain in the region of the carotid that radiates to the ear and jaw. It is made worse with palpation of the area overlying the carotid artery. Hyoid syndrome is characterized by sharp paroxysms of pain with swallowing or head turning. The pain radiates to the ear and the angle of the jaw, and can be reproduced with movement of the hyoid bone. In most cases, these unusual causes of ear, throat, and anterior neck pain are self-limited and produce no long-lasting harm to the patient. However, before they are diagnosed the clinician must rule out other pathologic processes that may harm the patient, because on a statistical basis they are much more common.

SUMMARY

Pain of the ear, nose, sinuses, and throat is commonly encountered in clinical practice. For the most part, the pathologic process responsible for the patient's symptoms is easily identifiable after the physician performs a targeted history and physical examination. Unfortunately, the nature of this anatomic region makes it possible for the most thorough physician to miss pathologic factors that may ultimately harm the patient. For this reason, the following rules for the treatment of ear, nose, sinus, and throat pain serve both the patient and the clinician well: (1) take a targeted history; (2) perform a careful, targeted physical examination; (3) heed the warning signs of serious disease, such as fever, constitutional symptoms, or weight loss; (4) image early and frequently if the diagnosis remains elusive; (5) perform laboratory tests that help identify "sick from well," such as erythrocyte sedimentation rate, hematology, and blood tests; (6) avoid attributing the patient's pain to idiopathic or psychogenic causes; and (7) always assume that you have missed the diagnosis.

REFERENCES

1. Waldman SD. Otalgia. Pain review. 1st edition. Philadelphia: Elsevier; 2009. p. 227–30.
2. Al-Sheikhli AR. Pain in the ear—with special reference to referred pain. J Laryngol Otol 1980;94:1433.
3. Waldman SD. Ramsey Hunt syndrome. In: Waldman SD, editor. Uncommon pain syndromes. 2nd edition. Philadelphia: Saunders; 2008. p. 25.
4. Khalak R, Roberts JK. Images in medicine—cauliflower ear. N Engl J Med 1996; 335:399.
5. Rapini RP, Warner NB. Relapsing polychondritis. Clin Dermatol 2006;24:482.
6. Beers SL, Abramo TJ. Otitis externa review. Pediatr Emerg Care 2004;20:254.
7. Kemppainen HO, Puhakka HJ, Laippala PJ, et al. Epidemiology and aetiology of middle ear cholesteatoma. Acta Otolaryngol 1999;119:568.
8. Davies PH, Benger JR. Foreign bodies in the nose and ear: a review of techniques for removal in the emergency department. J Accid Emerg Med 2000;17:91.
9. Bluestone CD. Clinical course, complications and sequelae of acute otitis media. Pediatr Infect Dis J 2000;19(Suppl 5):S37.
10. Nadol JB Jr, Eavey RD. Acute and chronic mastoiditis: clinical presentation, diagnosis, and management. Curr Clin Top Infect Dis 1995;15:204.
11. Thaller SR, De Silva A. Otalgia with a normal ear. Am Fam Physician 1987;36:129.
12. Eley CD, Gan VN. Picture of the month: folliculitis, furunculosis, and carbuncles. Arch Pediatr Adolesc Med 1997;151:625.
13. Kaliner MA, Osguthorpe JD, Fireman P. Sinusitis: bench to bedside: current findings, future directions. Otolaryngol Head Neck Surg 1997;116(6 Pt 2):S1.
14. Laine K, Maatta T, Varonen H. Diagnosing acute maxillary sinusitis in primary care: a comparison of ultrasound, clinical examination and radiography. Rhinology 1998;36:2.
15. Netscher DT, Spira M. Basal cell carcinoma: an overview of tumor biology and treatment. Plast Reconstr Surg 2004;113:74E.
16. Pensak ML, Gluckman JL, Shumrick KA. Parapharyngeal space tumors: an algorithm for evaluation and management. Laryngoscope 1994;104:1170.
17. Buttaravoli P. Pharyngitis: (sore throat). In: Buttaravoli P, editor. Minor emergencies. 2nd edition. New York: Elsevier; 2007. p. 156–61.
18. Kreisberg MK, Turner J. Dental causes of referred otalgia. Ear Nose Throat J 1987;66:398.
19. Beasley DJ, Amedee RG. Deep neck space infections. J La State Med Soc 1995; 147:181.
20. Yules RB. Differential diagnosis of referred otalgia. Eye Ear Nose Throat Mon 1967;46:587.
21. Som PM, Curtin HD. Lesions of the parapharyngeal space: role of MR imaging. Otolaryngol Clin North Am 1995;28:515.
22. Waldman SD. Eagle's syndrome. In: Waldman SD, editor. Uncommon pain syndromes. 2nd edition. Philadelphia: Saunders; 2008. p. 28.

Trigeminal Autonomic Cephalalgias Other than Cluster Headache

Stephen D. Silberstein, MD*, Nailia Vodovskaia, MD

KEYWORDS

- Trigeminal autonomic cephalalgia (TAC) • Paroxysmal hemicrania (PH) • SUNCT
- SUNA

KEY POINTS

- Trigeminal autonomic cephalalgias are a group of short-lasting primary headache disorders associated with autonomic symptoms.
- Paroxysmal hemicrania is a rare headache disorder similar to cluster headache, but attacks are shorter lasting, more frequent, more common in women, and are absolutely responsive to indomethacin.
- Short-lasting unilateral neuralgiform headache attacks with conjunctival injection and tearing (SUNCT) and short-lasting unilateral neuralgiform headache attacks with cranial autonomic symptoms (SUNA) are rare and unusual headache syndromes typified by a high frequency of severe, brief, unilateral attacks that usually occur in the distribution of the trigeminal nerve.
- SUNCT is a subtype of SUNA in which both conjunctival injection and tearing are present.
- SUNA differs from SUNCT in that autonomic symptoms are less prominent.

The trigeminal autonomic cephalalgias (TACs) are a group of headache disorders included in the third edition of the International Headache Society (IHS) classification.[1] The term was coined by Goadsby and Lipton[2] to reflect headache associated with excessive cranial parasympathetic autonomic reflex activation. TACs are a group of short-lasting primary headache disorders characterized by frequent, short-lasting attacks of severe, unilateral, orbital, supraorbital, or temporal pain associated with autonomic symptoms (conjunctival injection, lacrimation, nasal congestion, rhinorrhea, ptosis, and eyelid edema). Their symptoms often overlap, but each has characteristic features and different treatment responses.

Goadsby and Lipton[2] subdivided the TACs into cluster headache (episodic or chronic), episodic or chronic paroxysmal hemicranias (PHs), short-lasting unilateral

Jefferson Headache Center, 111 South 11th Street, Suite 8130, Philadelphia, PA 19107, USA
* Corresponding author.
E-mail address: stephen.silberstein@jefferson.edu

Med Clin N Am 97 (2013) 321–328
http://dx.doi.org/10.1016/j.mcna.2012.12.009 medical.theclinics.com

neuralgiform headache attacks with conjunctival injection and tearing (SUNCT), and short-lasting unilateral neuralgiform headache attacks with cranial autonomic symptoms (SUNA) (**Table 1**). The major discriminating feature for the different types of TACs is the duration and frequency of attacks. In general, forms with shorter-lived pain typically have a higher frequency of attacks (**Fig. 1**).

PH

PH is a rare headache disorder that has characteristics of pain and associated symptoms and signs similar to those of cluster headache, but they are shorter lasting, more frequent, more common in women, and are absolutely responsive to indomethacin. PH affects women more than men (ratio approximately 3:1) and the prevalence is approximately 2% that of cluster headache. PH has episodic and chronic subtypes (chronic is more common than episodic).[3,4]

Patients may evolve from the episodic to the chronic form of the illness. PH attacks are severe, unilateral, throbbing, boring, pulsatile, or stabbing pain in the distribution of the ophthalmic division of the trigeminal nerve.[5] The pain is associated with unilateral nasal stuffiness, lacrimation, conjunctival tearing, ptosis, and eyelid edema. PH attacks are less likely to cause agitation than cluster headache. The pain can also occur in the temporal, maxillary, frontal, retro-orbital, and occipital regions, and rarely it switches sides between attacks. Patients may have mild discomfort, soreness, or tenderness interictally, especially if attacks are frequent. This feature can make the differential diagnosis from hemicrania continua difficult. PH rarely may be associated with a typical migrainous aura.

Unlike patients with cluster headache, patients with PH usually sit quietly and hold their heads. Headaches average 13 minutes in duration and occur an average of 11 times throughout the day and night. Attacks may be triggered by flexing, rotating, or pressing the upper portion of the neck.[5] PH does not respond to standard cluster therapies and, by definition, must respond to indomethacin. PH usually begins in adulthood, with a mean age of 34 years and a range of 6 to 81 years. No family history of chronic or episodic PH has been reported (**Box 1**).[6]

Disorders that have been reported to mimic PH include circle of Willis aneurysms, parietal arteriovenous malformation, middle cerebral artery distribution and occipital infarction, frontal lobe tumor, gangliocytoma of the sella turcica, cavernous sinus meningioma, pituitary microadenoma, cerebral metastases of parotid epidermoid

Table 1
Differentiation between cluster headache, PH, and SUNCT/SUNA

Feature	Cluster Headache	PH	SUNCT/SUNA
Duration	15–180 min	2–30 min	5–240 s
Frequency (per d)	Every other day to 8	1–40	40–200
One-year prevalence (%)	0.1	0.05	0.1
Male/female ratio	4.3:1	1:1	1.5:1
Peak age onset	Third decade	Third to fourth decade	Fifth decade
Alcohol trigger	+++	+	−
Cutaneous trigger	−	−	+++
Circadian or circannual periodicity	Present	Absent	Absent

Modified from Nesbitt AD, Goadsby PJ. Cluster headache. BMJ 2012;344:e2407.

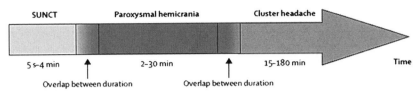

Fig. 1. Overlap between attack duration in TACs. The duration of each trigeminal autonomic cephalalgia is specified by the International Classification of Headache Disorders. (*Adapted from* Leone M, Bussone G. Pathophysiology of trigeminal autonomic cephalalgias. Lancet Neurol 2009;8(8):755–64.)

carcinoma, and Pancoast tumor. Because of this, magnetic resonance imaging (MRI) of the brain with attention to the pituitary region should be routinely performed in all patients with PH.[7]

The pathophysiology of PH is unknown. Patients with PH have decreased pain thresholds. They also have reduced corneal reflex thresholds and normal blink reflexes. Autonomic function studies, such as salivation, nasal secretion, and facial sweating, are normal. Patients with PH may have partial Horner syndrome. Cardiac events, such as bradycardia, bundle branch block, and atrial fibrillation, have been described in patients with PH during attacks. 15-H_2O positron emission tomography studies have shown activation in the posterior hypothalamus.[8] PH may coexist with trigeminal neuralgia, and PH-tic syndrome has been reported. Both components require individual treatment with indomethacin and carbamazepine. PH may also coexist with cough headache; both can be treated with indomethacin.[9,10]

Treatment

By definition, indomethacin in a daily dose of up to 225 mg (for at least 2 weeks) is effective in all published cases. Many patients need an initial high dose of indomethacin, following which the dose can be lowered. Indomethacin inhibits cyclooxygenase (predominantly cyclooxygenase-1), thus inhibiting synthesis of prostaglandin, a mediator of inflammation. It is not clear why indomethacin is more effective than other nonsteroidal antiinflammatory drugs, but it could be because of its central vasoconstrictive and analgesic properties, lowering of intracranial pressure, structural similarities to serotonin, or inhibition of metabolism of an active progesterone metabolite. Gastrointestinal side effects include discomfort and bleeding; these might be reduced by concomitant treatment with antacids, histamine H2 receptor antagonists, or proton pump inhibitors. Other nonsteroidal antiinflammatory drugs, gabapentin, and verapamil can be tried.

SUNCT AND SUNA

SUNCT and SUNA are among the rarest and most unusual headache syndromes; both are typified by an extremely high frequency (up to 200 attacks/d) of severe, brief, unilateral attacks that usually occur in the distribution of the trigeminal nerve. The syndrome was first described in 1978 (**Box 2**).[11,12]

SUNCT is a subtype of SUNA in which both conjunctival injection and tearing are present. SUNCT is more common in men, with a male/female ratio of 17:2 and age of onset from 10 to 77 years. Attacks are usually brief, lasting between 5 and 250 seconds.[13] Patients can have up to 30 episodes per hour; however, it is more common to have 5 to 6 episodes per hour. The unilateral pain is localized in the ophthalmic distribution of the trigeminal nerve, especially the orbital and periorbital

---

Box 1
International Classification of Headache Disorders, 3rd edition (ICHD-3) diagnostic criteria for PHs

3.2 PH

    A. At least 20 attacks fulfilling criteria B to E

    B. Attacks of severe unilateral pain lasting 2 to 30 minutes

    C. Attack frequency of more than 5 a day for more than half of the time, although periods with lower frequency may occur

    D. Pain associated with 1 or more of the following symptoms or signs on the pain side:

        1. Conjunctival injection, lacrimation, or both

        2. Nasal congestion, or rhinorrhea, or both

        3. Eyelid edema

        4. Forehead and facial sweating

        5. Forehead/facial flushing

        6. Sense of aural (ear) fullness

        7. Miosis, or ptosis, or both

    E. Headaches are prevented completely by indomethacin

    F. Not better accounted for by another diagnosis

3.2.1 Episodic PH

Description: occurs in periods lasting 7 days to 1 year separated by pain-free periods lasting 1 month or more

    Diagnostic criteria:

    A. All alphabetical headings of 3.2

    B. At least 2 bouts of headaches lasting (untreated patients) from 7 days to 1 year and separated by remissions of at least 1 month

3.2.2 Chronic PH

Description: attacks occur for more than 1 year without remission or with remissions lasting less than 1 month

    Diagnostic criteria:

    A. All alphabetical headings of 3.2

    B. Attacks recur over more than 1 year without remission periods or with remission periods lasting less than 1 month

From Headache Classification Subcommittee of the International Headache Subcommittee. The International Classification of Headache Disorders, 3rd edition. Cephalalgia, in press.

---

regions; it may radiate to other ipsilateral trigeminal divisions. The pain is stabbing, burning, pricking, piercing, shooting, or like an electric shock. Pain begins abruptly, reaching maximal intensity within seconds, and it continues at maximal intensity before rapidly resolving. Although attacks recur throughout the day, a bimodal distribution has been described, with increased frequency in the morning and afternoon/evening hours. Most patients are completely pain free between attacks, although some report a persistent, dull, interictal discomfort.[13–16] The conjunctival injection and lacrimation that occur during attacks are the most prominent autonomic features.

Box 2
ICHD-3 diagnostic criteria for SUNCT and SUNA

Diagnostic criteria

A. At least 20 attacks fulfilling criteria B to E

B. Attacks of short-lasting (1–600 s) unilateral head pain with the following features:

   a. Orbital, supraorbital, temporal, or other trigeminal distribution of moderate or severe pain

   b. Occurring:

      i. As single stabs

      ii. As groups of stabs

      iii. In a sawtooth pattern

C. Pain is accompanied ipsilaterally by 1 or more cranial autonomic symptoms:

   1. Conjunctival injection, lacrimation, or both

   2. Nasal congestion, or rhinorrhea, or both

   3. Eyelid edema

   4. Forehead and facial sweating

   5. Forehead/facial flushing

   6. Sense of aural (ear) fullness

   7. Miosis, or ptosis, or both

D. Attacks occur with a frequency of more than 1 per day for more than half the time when the disorder is active

E. Not better accounted for by another diagnosis

3.3.1 SUNCT

A. Fulfills criteria A to E of 3.3

B. Pain is accompanied ipsilaterally by both conjunctival injection and tearing

3.3.2 SUNA

A. Fulfills criteria A to E of 3.3

B. Fulfills 3.3 C

From Headache Classification Subcommittee of the International Headache Subcommittee. The International Classification of Headache Disorders, 3rd edition. Cephalalgia, in press.

Other less prominent autonomic stigmata include ipsilateral nasal congestion, rhinorrhea, forehead sweating, and eyelid edema.

Most patients can precipitate acute attacks by mechanical movement of the neck or by touching certain trigger zones within the trigeminal distribution (hair, forehead, face, nose, lips). Some patients can lessen or even abort attacks by moving their necks.

Secondary causes of SUNCT involving the posterior fossa and pituitary gland have been reported. Two reported patients had homolateral cerebellopontine angle arteriovenous malformation, whereas another had cavernous hemangioma of the brainstem. Cranial MRI is suggested in any suspected case of SUNCT.[7,17–19]

SUNA differs from SUNCT in that autonomic symptoms are less prominent. Both may be confused with trigeminal neuralgia (TN). Patients with SUNCT describe pain that begins in the ocular or forehead area, whereas TN pain is more common in the V2 area. Unlike patients with TN, most patients with SUNCT and SUNA have no refractory period.[14] One attack of SUNCT or SUNA may immediately follow another.

Cohen and colleagues[20] studied the phenotype of SUNCT and SUNA in a large series of patients (43 with SUNCT and 9 with SUNA). Three attack types were identified: stabs, groups of stabs, and sawtooth attacks. The mean duration of stabs was 58 seconds (1–600 seconds); stab groups, 396 seconds (10–1200 seconds); and sawtooth, 1160 seconds (5–12,000 seconds). The mean attack frequency was 59 attacks/d (2–600). Pain was orbital, supraorbital, or temporal in 38 (88%) patients with SUNCT and 7 (78%) patients with SUNA, and also occurred in the retro-orbital region; side, top, and back of head; second and third trigeminal divisions; teeth; neck; and ear. All patients with SUNCT had conjunctival injection and tearing. Two patients with SUNA had conjunctival injection, 4 had tearing, but none had both. Other cranial autonomic symptoms included nasal blockage, rhinorrhea, eyelid edema, facial sweating/flushing, and ear flushing. Cutaneous stimuli triggered attacks in 74% of patients with SUNCT but only 22% of patients with SUNA. Most (95% of patients with SUNCT and 89% of patients with SUNA) had no refractory period between attacks. Fifty-eight percent of patients with SUNCT and 56% of patients with SUNA were agitated with the attacks. The male/female ratio was 1.5:1 for total SUNCT and SUNA combined. When separated into SUNCT and SUNA, there was a higher male/female ratio in SUNCT (2:1), and almost the opposite ratio in SUNA (0.5:1) No patients with SUNA had attacks that could be triggered by touch, as opposed to 63% of patients with SUNCT, in whom touching the face could trigger attacks. Orbital phlebography was reported to be abnormal in patients with SUNCT, with narrowing of the superior ophthalmic vein homolateral to the pain. Forehead sweating is increased in patients with SUNCT, unlike patients with PH, who have normal forehead sweating. Bradycardia associated with SUNCT may indicate increased parasympathetic outflow. Transcranial Doppler and single-photon emission computed tomography studies are normal and have not shown changes in vasomotor activity or cerebral blood flow in patients with SUNCT. Functional MRI showed hypothalamic activation during attacks of SUNCT.[21–23] SUNCT probably results from an abnormality in the region of the hypothalamus, with subsequent trigeminovascular and cranial autonomic activation.

SUNCT is refractory to treatment. Because of the short-lasting nature of SUNCT and SUNA attacks, prophylaxis is a mainstay of treatment. The most effective means of short-term prevention is intravenous (IV) lidocaine. Matharu and colleagues[24] reported 4 cases of SUNCT in which IV lidocaine completely suppressed the headaches for the duration of the infusion. Two patients went on to have their symptoms controlled on topiramate (50–300 mg daily). Cohen[25] reviewed the effectiveness of treatment in 52 patients, 43 with SUNCT and 9 with SUNA. Of the 11 patients with SUNCT and 4 with SUNA who received IV lidocaine, 100% had a moderate to excellent effect. The patients with SUNA remained pain free for 2 days to 12 weeks after infusion. We have similar experience and think that treatment with lidocaine can suppress a severe exacerbation of SUNCT, and mexiletine may prevent recurrence. Lamotrigine is considered the first-line agent for long-term prevention. In case reports and observational studies, lamotrigine decreased the frequency or resulted in resolution of attacks. Lamotrigine should be initiated at a low dose (25 mg/d) and gradually increased to avoid serious adverse effects and to find the minimum effective dose. The risk of Stevens-Johnson syndrome, a dose-related adverse effect, can be minimized with gradual titration.[26] Some have suggested that topiramate, gabapentin, or carbamazepine might be effective. Invasive surgical procedures and hypothalamic stimulation should be reserved for refractory cases.

REFERENCES

1. Headache Classification Subcommittee of the International Headache Subcommittee. The International Classification of Headache Disorders, 3rd edition. Cephalalgia, in press.
2. Goadsby PJ, Lipton RB. A review of paroxysmal hemicranias, SUNCT syndrome and other short-lasting headaches with autonomic features, including new cases. Brain 1997;120:193–209.
3. Sjaastad O, Dale I. A new (?) clinical headache entity "chronic paroxysmal hemicrania" 2. Acta Neurol Scand 1976;54:140–59.
4. Kudrow L, Esperanz AP, Vijaya NN. Episodic paroxysmal hemicrania? Headache 1987;7:197–201.
5. Russell D, Vincent M. Chronic paroxysmal hemicrania. In: Olesen J, Tfelt-Hansen P, Welch KM, editors. The headaches. 2nd edition. Philadelphia: Lippincott Williams & Wilkins; 2000. p. 741–50.
6. Antonaci F, Sjaastad O. Chronic paroxysmal hemicrania (CPH): a review of the clinical manifestations. Headache 1989;29:648–56.
7. Goadsby PJ. Trigeminal autonomic cephalalgias: cluster headache and related conditions. In: Schapira AH, editor. Neurology and clinical neuroscience. Philadelphia: Mosby; 2007. p. 773–91.
8. Matharu MS, Cohen AS, Frackowiak RS, et al. Posterior hypothalamic activation in paroxysmal hemicrania. Ann Neurol 2006;59:535–45.
9. Hannerz J. Trigeminal neuralgia with chronic paroxysmal hemicrania: the CPH-tic syndrome. Cephalalgia 1993;13:361–4.
10. Caminero AB, Pareja JA, Dobato JL. Chronic paroxysmal hemicrania-tic syndrome. Cephalalgia 1998;18:159–61.
11. Sjaastad O, Russell D, Horven I, et al. Multiple neuralgiform unilateral headache attacks associated with conjunctival injection and appearing in clusters. A nosological problem. Proceedings of the Scandinavian Migraine Society. 1978. p. 31.
12. Sjaastad O, Saunte C, Salvesen R. Short-lasting unilateral neuralgiform headache attacks with conjunctival injection, tearing, sweating, and rhinorrhea. Cephalalgia 1989;9:147–56.
13. Pareja JA, Ming JM, Kruszewski P, et al. SUNCT syndrome: duration, frequency and temporal distribution of attacks. Headache 1996;36:161–5.
14. Pareja JA, Sjaastad O. SUNCT syndrome. A clinical review. Headache 1997;47:195–202.
15. Pareja JA, Sjaastad O. SUNCT syndrome in the female. Headache 1994;34:217–20.
16. Pareja JA, Caballero V, Sjaastad O. SUNCT syndrome. Status-like pattern. Headache 1996;36:622–4.
17. Bussone G, Leone M, Volta GD, et al. Short-lasting unilateral neuralgiform headache attacks with tearing and conjuctival injection: the first symptomatic case. Cephalalgia 1991;11:123–7.
18. De Benedittis G. SUNCT syndrome associated with cavernous angioma of the brain stem. Cephalalgia 1996;16:503–6.
19. Morales F, Mostacero E, Marta J, et al. Vascular malformation of the cerebellopontine angle associated with SUNCT syndrome. Cephalalgia 1994;14:301–2.
20. Cohen AS, Matharu MS, Goadsby PJ. Short-lasting unilateral neuralgiform headache attacks with conjunctival injection and tearing (SUNCT) or cranial autonomic features (SUNA)—a prospective clinical study of SUNCT and SUNA. Brain 2006;129:2746–60.

21. May A, Bahra A, Buchel C, et al. Functional magnetic resonance imaging in spontaneous attacks of SUNCT: short-lasting neuralgiform headache with conjunctival injection and tearing. Ann Neurol 1999;46:791–4.
22. Cohen AS, Matharu MS, Kalisch R, et al. Functional MRI in SUNCT shows differential hypothalamic activation with increasing pain. Cephalalgia 2004;24:1098–9.
23. Sprenger T, Valet M, Platzer S, et al. SUNCT: bilateral hypothalamic activation during headache attacks and resolving of symptoms after trigeminal decompression. Pain 2005;113:422–6.
24. Matharu MS, Cohen AS, Goadsby PJ. SUNCT syndrome responsive to intravenous lidocaine. Cephalalgia 2004;24:985–92.
25. Cohen AS. Short-lasting unilateral neuralgiform headache attacks with conjunctival injection and tearing. Cephalalgia 2007;27:824–32.
26. Rosselli JL, Karpinski JP. The role of lamotrigine in the treatment of short-lasting unilateral neuralgiform headache attacks with conjunctival injection and tearing syndrome. Ann Pharmacother 2011;45:108–13.

Giant Cell Arteritis

Corey W. Waldman, MD[a], Steven D. Waldman, MD, JD[b],*,
Reid A. Waldman[b]

KEYWORDS

- Giant cell • Arteritis • Artery • Erythrocyte sedimentation rate

KEY POINTS

- Pain on chewing, from claudication of the jaw muscles, occurs in up to two-thirds of patients suffering from giant cell arteritis.
- The mean age of onset of the symptoms of giant cell arteritis is approximately 70 years, with the condition being rare in those younger than 50 years.
- Women are affected about 3 times as often as men.
- The most common symptom of giant cell arteritis is headache, which is present in more than two-thirds of patients.

THE CLINICAL SYNDROME

Key clinical features of giant cell arteritis (GCA) are as follows:

1. A wide range of symptoms is seen, but most patients have clinical findings related to the involved arteries.
2. Frequent features include fatigue, headaches, jaw claudication, loss of vision, scalp tenderness, polymyalgia rheumatic (PMR), and aortic arch syndrome (decreased or absent peripheral pulses, discrepancies of blood pressure, arterial bruits).
3. Unlike other forms of vasculitis, GCA rarely involves the skin, kidneys, and lungs.
4. The erythrocyte sedimentation rate (ESR) is usually increased but may infrequently be normal.

The mean age of onset is approximately 70 years; the condition is rare in those younger than 50 years. Women are affected about 3 times as often as men. The onset can be dramatic but is usually insidious. The constitutional symptoms, including fever, anorexia, weight loss, and depression, are present in most patients, may be an early or even an initial finding, and can lead to a delay in diagnosis. Patients may present with

Large portions of this text were originally published in Hazleman B. Giant Cell Arteritis. In: Waldman SD, editor. Pain Management. 2nd Edition. Chapter 52: Elsevier; 2011. p. 476–81.
[a] Krieger Eye Institute At Sinai, 2411 West Belvedere Avenue, Baltimore, USA; [b] School of Medicine, University of Missouri-Kansas City, 2411 Holmes, Kansas City, Missouri, MO 64108, USA
* Corresponding author.
E-mail address: sdwaldmanmd@gmail.com

a pyrexia of unknown origin and be subjected to many investigations. The condition causes a wide range of symptoms, but most patients have clinical features related to the affected arteries. Common features include headache and tenderness of the scalp, particularly around the temporal and occipital arteries.

The most common symptom of GCA is headache, which is present in more than two-thirds of patients. It usually begins early in the course of the disease and may be the presenting symptom. The pain is severe and localized to the temple. However, it may be occipital or be less defined and precipitated by brushing the hair. Headache can be severe even when the arteries are clinically normal and, conversely, may subside even when the disease remains active. The nature of the pain varies; some patients describe it as shooting, and others as more like a steady ache. Scalp tenderness is common, particularly around the temporal and occipital arteries, and may disturb sleep. Tender spots, or nodules, or even small skin infarcts may be present for several days. The vessels are thickened, tender, and nodular with absent or reduced pulsation. Sometimes they are red and clearly visible (**Fig. 1**).

Visual disturbances have been described in 25% to 50% of cases, although the incidence of visual loss is thought to be lower, about 6% to 10% in most series, which is probably the result of earlier recognition and treatment.[1-6] Visual symptoms are an ophthalmic emergency; if they are identified and treated urgently, blindness is usually preventable. The variety of ocular lesions essentially results from occlusion of the various orbital or ocular arteries. Blindness is the most serious, and irreversible, feature. The visual loss is usually sudden, painless, and permanent; it may vary from mistiness of vision or involvement of a part of the visual field, to complete blindness. The second eye is at risk of involvement if the patient is not treated aggressively. Involvement of the second eye can occur within 24 hours. Blindness may be the initial presentation in cases of GCA, but it tends to follow other symptoms by several weeks or months.

The incidence of various ocular manifestations given in the literature varies widely because the incidence depends on several factors, the most important of which is how early the diagnosis of GCA is established and the treatment started. It also depends on the rigor with which cases are diagnosed. The most common cases are optic nerve ischemic lesions (**Fig. 2**). These lesions are usually anterior and are associated with partial or, more frequently, complete visual loss. They can occasionally be posterior, which can lead to partial or complete loss. Extraocular mobility disorders are usually transient and not associated with visual loss. Pupillary abnormalities can be seen as a result of visual loss. Cerebral ischemic lesions producing visual loss

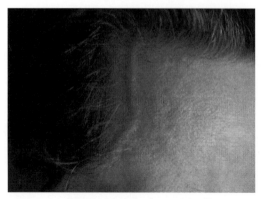

Fig. 1. Clinical appearance suggesting temporal arteritis. (*From* Masson C. Therapeutic approach to giant cell arteritis. Joint Bone Spine 2012;79(3):219–27.)

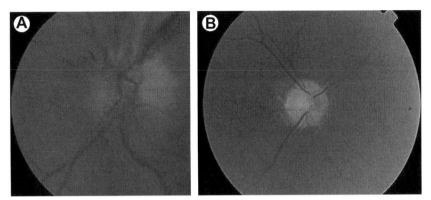

Fig. 2. The optic disc in patients with GCA and visual loss caused by anterior ischemic optic neuropathy, in the early acute phase (*A*) and after 3 months of prednisone therapy (*B*). (*A*) Optic disc edema and a flame-shaped hemorrhage are shown. (*B*) Optic atrophy is shown. (*From* Salvarani C, Cantini F, Hunder GG. Polymyalgia rheumatica and giant-cell arteritis. Lancet 2008;372(9634):234–45.)

are rare, as are anterior segment ischemic lesions and choroidal infarcts. Retinal ischemic lesions can affect the central retinal artery, which is associated with severe visual loss. The cilioretinal artery can be occluded but is invariably associated with anterior ischemic optic neuropathy (AION).

Pain on chewing, from claudication of the jaw muscles, occurs in up to two-thirds of patients. Tingling in the tongue, loss of taste, and pain in the mouth and throat can also occur, presumably as a result of vascular insufficiency. The widespread nature of the vasculitis has been mentioned previously. Clinical evidence of large artery involvement is present in 10% to 15% of cases, and, in some instances, aortic dissection and rupture occur.

Less common features of GCA include hemiparesis, peripheral neuropathy, deafness, depression, and confusion. Involvement of the coronary arteries may lead to myocardial infarction. Aortic regurgitation and congestive cardiac failure may also occur. Abnormalities of thyroid and liver function are well described. An association between carpal tunnel syndrome and PMR has been noted by several investigators. Local corticosteroid injection or surgical decompression is sometimes necessary.

RELATIONSHIP BETWEEN PMR AND GCA

In recent years, GCA and PMR have increasingly been considered to be closely related conditions.[7,8] The two syndromes form a spectrum of diseases and affect the same types of patients. The conditions may occur independently or may occur in the same patient, either together or separately.

In patients with PMR who have no symptoms or signs of GCA, positive temporal biopsy results are found in 10% to 15%. Those investigators who wish to preserve the identity of the two diseases base their argument on the latter figure and on the failure to find evidence of arteritis in many patients followed for many years with polymyalgia. In contrast, many similarities are seen between the two conditions. The age and gender distributions are similar, the biopsy findings show an identical pattern, and the laboratory features are similar, although many are nonspecific inflammatory changes. In addition, similarity is found in the myalgia, in the associated systemic features, and in the response to corticosteroid therapy.

The onset of myalgic symptoms may precede, coincide with, or follow those of the arteritic symptoms. No difference has been found between the characteristics of those patients with myalgia with positive biopsy results and those with no histologic evidence of arteritis. Mild aching and stiffness may persist for months after other features of GCA have remitted. There is little evidence to suggest that the musculo-skeletal symptoms are related to vasculitis. Many patients with GCA do not have PMR, even when large vessels are involved. In addition, the finding of joint swelling in some patients and the production of pain with the injection of 5% saline solution into the acromioclavicular, sternoclavicular, and manubriosternal joints suggests that PMR in some patients may be a particular form of proximal synovitis.

CLINICAL TESTING

One of the most frequently performed diagnostic tests in suspected cases of GCA is temporal artery biopsy. The choice of patients for biopsy depends on local circum-stances, but a pragmatic policy is selection of only patients with suspected GCA (not those with obvious clinical features). Patients with PMR alone need to be moni-tored carefully for development of clinical GCA and do not need a biopsy.

One-third of patients with signs and symptoms of cranial arteritis may have negative temporal artery biopsy results, which may be the result of the localized involvement of arteries in the head and neck. Temporal artery biopsy may show arteritis even after 14 days of corticosteroid treatment, so biopsy may be worthwhile for up to 2 weeks of treatment. However, the biopsy should be obtained as soon as possible, and treatment of suspected GCA should not be delayed simply to allow a biopsy to be performed.

Clinicians vary in their approach to temporal artery biopsy. Some think that it emphasizes the value of a positive histologic diagnosis, especially months or years later when side effects of the steroid treatment have developed. Others think that a high false-negative rate diminishes the value of the procedure. In most instances, the high false-negative rate can be attributed to the focal nature of involvement of the superficial temporal artery by the inflammatory process.

The histologic appearance of GCA is one of the most distinctive of vascular disor-ders. The dense granulomatous inflammatory infiltrates that characterize the acute stages of the disease resemble those of Takayasu arteritis, but the clinicopathologic features in patients with positive temporal artery biopsy results are diagnostic. The arteritis is histologically a panarteritis with giant cell granuloma formation, often in close proximity to a disrupted internal elastic lamina. Large and medium-sized arteries are affected; the involvement is patchy, and skip lesions are often found. Most patients with skip lesions have normal arteries to palpation but do not have a benign disease.

The gross features are not characteristic. The vessels are enlarged and nodular and have little or no lumen. Thrombosis often develops at sites of active inflammation. Later, these areas may recanalize. The lumen is narrowed by intimal proliferation, which is a common finding in arteries and may result from advancing age, nearby chronic inflammation, or low blood flow. The adventitia is usually invaded by mononu-clear, and occasionally polymorphonuclear, inflammatory cells, often cuffing the vasa vasorum; here, fibrous proliferation is frequent. The changes in the media are domi-nated by the giant cells, which vary from small cells with 2 to 3 nuclei up to masses of 100 nm containing many nuclei. Invasion by mononuclear cells that resemble histio-cytes is found here. Fibrinoid necrosis is infrequent. Giant cells are not seen in all sections and, therefore, are not required for the diagnosis if other features are compat-ible. The more sections that are examined in the area of arteritis, the more likely it is that giant cells will be found.

Corticosteroids reduce the inflammatory cell infiltrate so temporal artery biopsy should, if possible, be performed before treatment is started. Therapy should not be delayed until a biopsy has been performed. Involvement of the aorta and its branches, the abdominal vessels, and the coronary arteries has been described. GCA as a cause of aortic dissection has been recorded rarely at autopsy, and most exceptionally during life, which probably reflects the low incidence of aortic involvement in GCA. Most patients have a history of hypertension or features of hypertensive disease at autopsy.

The ESR is usually greatly increased and provides a useful means of monitoring treatment, although some increase of the ESR may occur in otherwise healthy elderly people. A normal ESR is occasionally found in patients with active biopsy-proven disease. Repeated measurements may show increased ESRs after an initial normal value.

Anemia, usually of a mild hypochromic type, is common and resolves without specific treatment, but more marked normochromic anemia occasionally occurs and may be a presenting symptom. Leukocyte and differential counts are generally normal; platelet counts are also usually normal but may be increased. Protein electrophoresis may show a nonspecific increase in $alpha_2$ globulin, with less frequent increase of $alpha_1$ globulin and gamma globulin. Quantification of acute-phase proteins and $alpha_1$-antitrypsin, orosomucoid, haptoglobin, and C-reactive protein (CRP) are no more helpful than the ESR in the assessment of disease activity.

Abnormalities of thyroid and liver function have also been well described. In a retrospective survey of 59 cases of GCA, 5 patients with hyperthyroidism were identified.[9] The arteritis followed the thyrotoxicosis by intervals of 4 to 15 years in 3 cases, and it occurred simultaneously in 2. In 250 patients with autoimmune thyroid disease, 7 cases of PMR or GCA were identified. All cases occurred in women older than 60 years, for a prevalence rate of 9.3% in this age group.[10–13]

Increased serum values for alkaline phosphatase were found in up to 70% of patients with PMR, and transaminases in some cases were mildly increased. Liver biopsies have shown portal and intralobular inflammation with focal liver cell necrosis and small epithelioid cell granuloma. The pathologic significance of these abnormalities is unclear.

TREATMENT

Corticosteroids are mandatory in the treatment of GCA; they reduce the incidence of complications, such as blindness, and rapidly relieve symptoms. Nonsteroidal antiinflammatory drugs (NSAIDs) lessen the painful symptoms, but they do not prevent arteritic complications. The response to corticosteroids is usually dramatic and occurs within days. Corticosteroid treatment has improved the quality of life for patients, although no evidence shows that therapy reduces the duration of the disease. A fear of vascular complications in patients with positive biopsy results often leads to the use of high doses of corticosteroids. Recent studies have emphasized the importance of adopting a cautious and individual treatment schedule and have highlighted the efficacy of lower doses of prednisolone.

At first, the corticosteroids should be given at a sufficient dosage to control the disease and then be maintained at the lowest dosage that controls the symptoms and lowers the ESR. In patients with GCA, corticosteroids should preferably be given after the diagnosis has been confirmed histologically. However, when GCA is strongly suspected, there should be no delay in starting therapy because the artery biopsy will still show inflammatory changes for several days after corticosteroids have been started and the result is unlikely to alter therapeutic decisions. If the temporal artery (or other artery) biopsy shows no arteritis but the suspicion of disease is strong, corticosteroid treatment should be started. The danger is delay in therapy because blindness may occur at any time.

Few clinical trials exist to help determine the correct initial dose. Most clinicians have strong views on the dose needed, but some views are based on tradition and anecdote. The recommended initial dose for PMR/GCA varies from 10 mg to 100 mg prednisolone daily. Intravenous corticosteroids are occasionally used if there are visual complications. In practice, most clinicians use 10 to 20 mg prednisolone daily to treat PMR and 40 to 60 mg for GCA because of the higher risk of arteritic complications in cases of GCA. Some ophthalmologists suggest an initial dose of at least 60 mg because they have seen blindness occur at a lower dose. However, this has to be balanced against the potential complication of high dosage in this older age group. Patients should be advised that, although they are taking a maintenance dose of steroids, any sudden exacerbation of symptoms, particularly sudden visual deterioration, necessitates an immediate increase in dose.

Glucocorticoid therapy is adequate for most patients with GCA but, in those with long-standing glucocorticoid-resistant disease and those at risk of glucocorticoid-related adverse events, glucocorticoid-sparing agents should be considered (these include methotrexate and tumor necrosis factor α [TNFα] blockers).

Methotrexate seems to be effective in GCA but does not have a rapid onset of action and cannot be recommended as a replacement for glucocorticoids at disease onset. TNFα inhibition is to some extent effective in long-standing, refractory GCA but is not effective in new-onset GCA.[14]

PROGNOSIS

Rapid reduction or withdrawal of corticosteroids has been reported to contribute to deaths in patients with GCA. However, complications are rare, and the activity of the disease seems to decline steadily. Relapses are more likely during the initial 18 months of treatment and within 1 year of withdrawal of corticosteroids. There is no reliable method of predicting those most at risk, but arteritic relapses in patients who present with pure PMR are unusual. Temporal artery biopsy does not seem helpful in predicting outcome.

Controversy exists over the expected duration of the disease. Most European studies within the last 20 years report that between one-third and one-half of the patients are able to discontinue corticosteroids after 2 years of treatment. Studies from the Mayo Clinic in the United States have reported a shorter duration of disease for both PMR (11 months was the median duration of treatment, and three-quarters of patients had stopped taking corticosteroids by 2 years) and GCA (most patients had stopped taking corticosteroids within 2 years).[15] The consensus is that stopping treatment is feasible from 2 years onward.

Patients who are unable to reduce the dosage of prednisolone because of recurring symptoms or who have serious corticosteroid-related side effects pose particular problems. Drugs such as azathioprine and methotrexate have not been shown to exert a corticosteroid-sparing effect in corticosteroid-resistant cases of PMR/GCA.

Between one-fifth and one-half of patients may experience serious treatment-related side effects. Serious side effects are significantly related to high initial doses, maintenance doses, cumulative doses, and increased duration of treatment. Side effects can be minimized with low doses of prednisolone whenever possible.

In elderly people, corticosteroid treatment carries the risk of increasing osteoporosis. Glucocorticoids have more effect on the spine than on the femur. Bisphosphonates, such as etidronate and alendronate, have been shown to be useful in retarding bone loss in the setting of prolonged corticosteroid use.

SUMMARY

GCA is the prime medical emergency in ophthalmology because it may result in loss of vision in 1 or both eyes. This vision loss is preventable if patients are diagnosed early and treated immediately with high doses of corticosteroids.

REFERENCES

1. Horton BT, Magath TB, Brown GE. An undescribed form of arteritis of the temporal vessels. Mayo Clin Proc 1932;7:700.
2. Paulley JW, Hughes JP. Giant cell arteritis, or arteritis of the aged. Br Med J 1960; 2:1562.
3. Rahman W, Rahman FZ. Giant cell (temporal) arteritis: an overview and update. Surv Ophthalmol 2005;50:415.
4. Salvarani C, Gabriel SE, O'Fallon WM, et al. Epidemiology of polymyalgia rheumatica in Olmsted County, Minnesota, 1970-1991. Arthritis Rheum 1995;38:369.
5. Nordborg C, Johansson H, Petursdottir V, et al. The epidemiology of biopsy-positive giant cell arteritis: special reference to changes in the age of the population. Rheumatology 2003;42:549.
6. Ostberg G. An arteritis with special reference to polymyalgia arteritica. Acta Pathol Microbiol Scand 1973;237(Suppl):1.
7. Cantini F, Niccoli L, Storri L, et al. Are polymyalgia rheumatica and giant cell arteritis the same disease? Semin Arthritis Rheum 2004;33:294.
8. Gonzalez-Gay MA. Giant cell arteritis and polymyalgia rheumatica: two different but often overlapping conditions. Semin Arthritis Rheum 2004;33:289.
9. Thomas RD, Croft DN. Thyrotoxicosis and giant cell arteritis. Br Med J 1974;2: 408.
10. Nicholson GC, Gutteridge DH, Carroll WM, et al. Auto-immune thyroid disease and giant cell arteritis: a review, case report, and epidemiological study. Aust N Z J Med 1984;14:487.
11. Ly KH, Régent A, Tamby MC, et al. Pathogenesis of giant cell arteritis: more than just an inflammatory condition? Autoimmun Rev 2010;9(10):635-45.
12. Weyand CM, Tetzlatt N, Bjornsson J, et al. Disease patterns and tissue cytokine profiles in giant cell arteritis. Arthritis Rheum 1997;40:19.
13. Blockmans D, Condyzer W, Vanderschueren S, et al. Relationship between fluorodeoxyglucose uptake in the large vessels and late aortic diameter in giant cell arteritis. Rheumatology (Oxford) 2008;47:1179.
14. Salvarani C, Pipitone N, Buiardi L, et al. Do we need treatment with tumour necrosis factor blockers for giant cell arteritis. Ann Rheum Dis 2008;67:577.
15. Proven A, Gabriel SE, Orces C, et al. Glucocorticoid therapy in giant cell arteritis: duration and adverse outcomes. Arthritis Rheum 2003;49:703.

Medication Overuse Headaches

Bernard M. Abrams, MD

KEYWORDS

- Medication overuse headache • Chronic daily headaches • Triptans • Ergots
- Opioids • Combination analgesics • Detoxification • Prophylactic medications

KEY POINTS

- Overuse of any class of drugs, Triptans, ergots, opioids, simple, or combination analgesics used to treat acute headaches, especially migraine, can lead to the development of medication overuse headache.
- People suffering from primary headache types, such as migraine or tension-type headache, are at higher risk to develop chronic headache following the overuse of acute headache drugs.
- Treatment of medication overuse headache requires withdrawal as an initial step, coincident initiation of preventive treatment, a multidisciplinary setting, and includes education of patients.
- Treatment strategies must include decisions on withdrawal of medications on an outpatient or in hospital setting and a detoxification plan that minimizes patient discomfort.

Medication overuse for headaches and subsequent medication overuse headache (MOH) is a growing problem worldwide. Epidemiologic data suggest that up to 4% of the population overuse analgesics and other drugs for the treatment of pain conditions such as migraine and that about 1% of the general population in Europe, North America, and Asia have MOH.[1] MOH is far easier to prevent than cure, and any agent used in the acute treatment of headaches can, with overuse, initiate MOH. These include the newer agents such as the Triptans as well as older agents including ergots, combination drugs, especially with barbiturates, opioids, and others to be detailed below. The recent admonition to treat headaches, especially migraines, early has compounded the problem and encouraged more frequent use of headache abortive medications, especially the Triptans, when beginning headaches may or may not evolve into full-blown headaches. Patients, eager to avoid full-blown headaches, especially disabling migraines, may subscribe to the "more is better" medical philosophy and become prone to MOH.

The author has nothing to disclose.
Department of Neurology, University of Missouri-Kansas City, School of Medicine, Kansas City, MO 64106, USA
E-mail address: babrams@kc.rr.com

Med Clin N Am 97 (2013) 337–352
http://dx.doi.org/10.1016/j.mcna.2012.12.007
0025-7125/13/$ – see front matter © 2013 Elsevier Inc. All rights reserved.

medical.theclinics.com

CRITERIA FOR DIAGNOSIS

MOH previously known as rebound headache, drug-induced headache, or medication-misuse headache has the following diagnostic criteria[2,3]:

A. Headache present for more than 15 days per month fulfilling criteria C and D.
B. Regular overuse of 1 or more drugs that can be taken for acute and/or symptomatic treatment of headache for more than 3 months.
C. Headache has developed or markedly worsened during medication overuse.
D. Headache resolves or reverts to its previous pattern within 2 months after discontinuation of overused medication.

The criteria were further revised in 2006 to remove the requirement for cessation of the headache or reversion to baseline after 2 months.[4]

HISTORY

Although credit for describing MOH first has been given to Horton and Peters in 1963,[5] Peters himself had presaged the association of ergot withdrawal and headache in 1951.[6] As Isler points out, "warnings against worsening of headaches by "too strong drugs" are found at least from the seventeenth century onward (Maxwell 1679)."[7]

PLACE IN CLASSIFICATION

From the seemingly endless number of headache entities, the International Classification of Headache Disorders (ICHD-2) in 1988,[8] updated in the year 2004,[2] offers a new understanding of headache disorders. It is the key to the diagnosis and treatment of headaches. It divides headaches into primary and secondary with 4 primary headache categories and 8 secondary headache categories. A primary headache disorder is not due to another condition, whereas a secondary headache disorder is due to another identifiable condition such as a brain tumor.
The primary headache disorders are

1. Migraine
2. Tension-type headache
3. Cluster and other trigeminal autonomic cephalgias
4. Other primary headaches

The secondary headache disorders are

1. Head and neck trauma
2. Cranial or cervical vascular disorders
3. Nonvascular intracranial disorders
4. Substance abuse or withdrawal disorders
5. Infection
6. Disorders of homeostasis
7. Disorders of the cranium, neck, eyes, nose, sinuses, teeth, mouth, or other facial or cranial structures
8. Psychiatric

The distinction between primary and secondary headaches is the key. There are 2 goals for any headache evaluation:

1. The recognition of primary headache syndromes for which treatment is available.
2. The recognition of secondary syndromes, which may constitute a threat to life or function.

One can best understand MOH in the context of chronic daily headache of which it is a subset. Its position as a primary or secondary headache depends on the evolution of the headache and whether one considers MOH as a separate entity or a natural evolution of a primary headache disorder. Although the diagnosis and treatment do not change substantially, because it is a headache with a known cause, it tends to be classified as secondary headache disorder by some. In 1996, Silberstein and colleagues[9] published a proposed classification of chronic primary headaches defined as those of greater than 4 hours duration and occurring 15 days per month or more. The term "chronic daily headache" was used for this classification. This system looked at the longitudinal evolution of the headache syndrome and included the following entities: (1) transformed migraine: chronic headache evolving from intermittent migraine, (2) chronic tension-type headache: chronic headache evolving from intermittent tension-type headache, (3) new daily persistent headache: a primary headache that is chronic from onset, and (4) hemicrania continua. These 4 entities were all modified by the presence or absence of medication overuse, which is classified as a secondary headache with occasional migraine by the ICHD-2. The problem of medication overuse has been a major issue complicating the understanding of chronic daily headache syndromes because efforts to define and classify headache in this area has begun.[10,11]

A major problem of classification that arises is whether MOH is a separate entity or a part of the chronic daily headache syndromes as suggested by the Silberstein-Lipton classification. The ICHD-2 classifies MOH as an organic headache that is superimposed on the syndromes of chronic daily headache, whereas the Silberstein-Lipton criteria consider MOH to be a part of chronic daily headache. Even recent publications have queried whether chronic migraine plus MOH are two entities or one.[12]

OFFENDING AGENTS

Any agent used to treat acute headaches may cause MOH. The duration of treatment and frequency vary in different studies. The ICHD-2 classification for MOH suggests that a medication be regularly overused for more than equal to 3 months for acute/symptomatic treatment and goes on to enumerate the various drugs as ergotamines, Triptans, analgesics, opioids, combination analgesics, combinations of acute medications, and other medications.

Although the emphasis is on ergotamines, Triptans, opioids, and combination drugs (most notably containing caffeine or a barbiturate), a complete list is exhaustive with simple analgesics acetaminophen, aspirin, and combination drugs including caffeine (Excedrin); nonsteroidal antiinflammatory drugs (NSAIDs); butalbital and its congeners; minor narcotics including codeine, oxycodone, hydrocodone, and, until recently, propoxyphene; as well as major narcotics meperidine, morphine and narcotic agonist/antagonist drugs butorphanol and nalbuphine.[13]

Styles in MOH change as new drugs are developed and when Triptans were developed, the incidence of MOH from ergots dropped markedly. As new Triptans came on the market, generally cases of MOH were reported a year after a drug had been approved.[1] The diagnostic criteria in the ICHD-II[14,15] listed ergotamines as requiring 10 days per month for more than 3 months, Triptans more than 15 days per month (with additional requirements generally satisfying the criteria for the diagnosis of migraine headache) or 10 days per month for more than 3 months, simple analgesics for 15 days per month for more than 3 months, opioids for 10 days per month for more than 3 months, and combination analgesics for 10 days per month for more than

3 months. A prospective study of 96 patients investigated the characteristics of MOH in relation to different drugs.[16] In this study, done between 1999 and 2001, Triptan overuse caused MOH in many more cases than ergot overuse. The delay between the starting of drug use and the development of daily headache was shortest for Triptans (1–7 years), longer for ergots (2–7 years), and longest for analgesics (4–8 years). The intake frequency (single doses per month) was lowest for Triptans (18 doses), higher for ergots (37 doses), and highest for analgesics (114 doses). Triptans do not only cause a different set of clinical features as will be seen in the clinical picture section but also causes MOH faster and with lower doses than other groups of drugs.[1] A somewhat contradictory view of the relative risk of various acute medications was advanced by Tepper and Tepper[17] from the Cleveland Clinic who stated "a pivotal study[18] found "that butalbital combinations were most likely to cause medication overuse headache," needing to be taken on merely 5 or more days per month to cause MOH in migraineurs. Opioids caused MOH it if taken 8 or more days per month and Triptans if taken10 or more days per month. NSAIDs actually protected against transformation to daily headache if used 5 or fewer days per month but caused MOH if used 10 or more days per month. This is especially ironic because the Food and Drug Administration has approved a sumatriptan-naproxen combination for abortive therapy for migraine, which appears rational in light of secondary allodynia induced after the initial state of migraine cephalgias.

Thus, the investigators stated, "there was a hierarchy of risk, with butalbital being the worst, opioids in the middle, and NSAIDs and Triptans the least risky. None of the agents had to be taken daily to trigger medication overuse headache." Other studies have given different proportions and relative risks, but the overriding conclusion is that all acute headache medications can cause MOH and overuse is to be avoided.

CLINICAL PICTURE

The clinical manifestations of MOH include any combination of (1) gradually worsening headache; (2) increasing analgesic or Triptan use; (3) a particularly strong headache when analgesics are discontinued; and (4) failure of preventive medication to modify the headaches. The onset of MOH is typically insidious with progression to a rebound-withdrawal headache pattern over months or even years. The changes in headache occurrence are usually not recognized by the patient and sometimes the treating physician because related to frequent usage of symptomatic medication, and patients are usually resistant to the idea that the symptomatic medication is, in fact, the cause of the worsening headache problem. Analgesic-overuse headaches may be accompanied by behavioral abnormalities and medication-seeking behavior.

The character of the headache in the MOH syndrome is usually tension-type headache. Triptan overuse, however, may lead to MOH with features of migraine without aura in migraine sufferers. Patients overusing Triptans only appeared to develop frequent migraine-like headache attacks, whereas patients who overused Triptans and analgesics reported continuous headache superimposed with migraine attacks. Unlike patients with MOH caused by ergot or analgesic overuse, patients with migraine (but not those with tension-type headache) with Triptan-induced headache did not describe the typical tension-type daily headache, but rather a migraine-like daily headache (a unilateral, pulsating headache with autonomic disturbances) or a significant increase in migraine attack frequency.[1] Variable pain location is a particular characteristic of MOH. Although the location may differ from day to day (front or back, rostral or caudal, unilateral or bilateral), it is the quantity not the quality or location of the headaches that suggests the diagnosis.[17]

For patients with chronic (formerly transformed) migraine and superimposed MOH, there may be a combination of tension-type headache and migraine features resulting from overuse of any of the earlier mentioned combinations. "Little" headaches usually manifest the appearance of tension-type headaches, whereas the "big" headaches often retain features of migraine. As the MOH becomes well established, the patient may begin to note a cycling of headache pain associated with dosing of symptomatic medication. Predictably, the headaches come in the early morning or awaken the patient from sleep, and this may be because of variable drug withdrawal and indicates a drug-dependent rhythm.[17] Longer intervals since the last dose of the MOH-inducing agent produce a more severe headache. Usually the pain, photophobia, and phono-phobia are prominent, whereas other features usually seen in migraine may be less prominent. Gastrointestinal and neurologic symptoms accompanying the headache are usually much less evident. The pattern of "big" and "little" headaches may become blunted. Sudden withdrawal of the MOH-inducing agent will usually precipitate a severe or even disabling headache.

Less frequently recognized manifestations are neck pain, depression and anxiety, nonrestorative sleep, and vasomotor instability.[17]

MOH frequently involves the neck, and patients often seek and receive treatments such as muscle relaxants or injections to the neck. When patients are weaned from their acute migraine medications, the neck pain will often subside but the neck pain can recur periodically with their remaining, now-episodic acute migraines. Neck pain associated with MOH is not usually a sign of a primary neck disorder but is a symptom of MOH itself. Physical therapy and other modalities designed to relieve neck pain are usually minimally effective. Although depression and anxiety are commonly seen in episodic migraine, they appear to be more common with MOH. Treatment of the depression or anxiety does not restore an episodic pattern of migraine; weaning from the overused medications remains the most important inter-vention. "A frequent clinical error is to diagnose and treat the psychiatric issues without recognizing medication overuse as the primary problem."[17]

Nonrestorative sleep is frequently reported by patients with MOH. This is often because of the caffeine contained in combination analgesics or excessive dietary caffeine intake, but it may also be part of the daily acute drug withdrawal syndrome or associated with the concomitant depression. Sleep often improves after weaning from the offending medications. The sleep disorder pain is not primary but a manifes-tation of MOH.

Autonomic features are commonly associated with MOH. Rhinorrhea, nasal stuffi-ness, and lacrimation are features of medication withdrawal, especially from opioids, and are frequently attributed to sinus disease or "sinus headaches."[17]

EPIDEMIOLOGY

As stated earlier, MOH has been termed a worldwide epidemic and estimated to affect approximately 1% of the population.[19] Cross-sectional, population-based, epidemio-logic studies indicate that chronic headache is common with prevalence between 2% and 5%, and the prevalence of chronic headache associated with MOH or probable MOH is about 1%. There is evidence that the overuse of analgesics and subsequent MOH is not only prevalent in Europe and North America but also a growing problem in Asian countries; in China and Taiwan the prevalence is the same as in Europe.

Any study of the epidemiology of MOH must begin with the concept that the majority are an evolution of primary headache entities, acute or episodic into their chronic form, for example, episodic migraine into chronic migraine. Diener and

Daholf[19] in a meta-analysis of 29 studies identified 65% of the patients reporting migraine as their primary headache, 27% of patients reporting tension-type headache as their primary headache, and 8% of patients reporting mixed or other headaches as their primary headache. Zeeberg and colleagues[20] described a prospective cohort of 216 patients with MOH from the Danish Headache Center. Twenty-one percent of them had migraine, 43% had migraine and tension-type headache, and 14% had another headache type. Median headache duration was 17 years. The most frequently overused drugs were combination analgesics (42%), followed by simple analgesics (29%), Triptans (20%), opioids (6%), and ergots (4%). Women were more prone to MOHs than men (3.5:1; 1533 women, 442 men). This ratio is slightly higher than would be expected from the gender differences in frequency of migraine. The mean duration of primary headache was 20.4 years. The mean admitted time of frequent drug intake was 10.3 years, and the mean duration of daily headache was 5.9 years. The mean time of frequent drug intake and chronic headache was much shorter for ergotamine and Triptans than for analgesics (**Fig. 1**).[18,21]

Children may also be affected, beginning in childhood or adolescence although precise data are not available. Most headache centers report that between 5% and 10% of the patients they follow-up fulfill the criteria of MOH. In a large population-based study,[18] 2.5% of patients who began with episodic migraine (headaches on fewer than 15 days per month) had "transformed migraine" (headaches on 15 or more days per month) 1 year later. The prevalence of chronic daily headache is almost 5% of the general population and may account for up to 70% of the initial diagnoses seen in headache centers. The closer a patient is to having 15 headaches per month, the more likely she or he will cross the line.[22,23] In a German study, observing patients for 1 year in a neurology clinic it was found that those starting the year with 6 to 9 headaches per month were 6.2 times more likely to develop chronic daily headache in the next year than those who began the year with 0 to 4 per month and those starting with 10 to 14 headaches per month were 20 times more likely to develop chronic headaches.

Patients taking chronic analgesics without headaches are far less prone to develop MOH. For example, patients who were consuming fairly large amounts of analgesics regularly for arthritis did not show an increased incidence of headache.[24,25]

ILLUSTRATIVE CASES
Case Report 1

A 48-year-old woman presented with migraine attacks almost daily for 2 years. She had no aura but she would have a headache the day before because of irritability

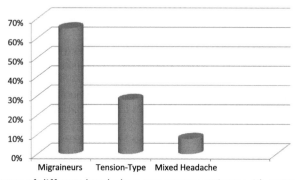

Fig. 1. Percentages of different headache types among patients with MOH.

and a craving for high carbohydrate foods. Her migraines started at 20 years of age. At first, her attacks were infrequent, but the attack frequency had increased over the last 10 years, culminating in her present state. She treated her migraine attacks with an oral Triptan, which initially was highly effective. About 4 years ago, her migraine attacks became longer, lasting up to 72 to 96 hours and becoming incapacitating. She missed substantial work until she was terminated from her job. She was taking 4 to 5 doses of Triptans per attack. At the time of presentation, she was averaging 25 doses of oral Triptans per month. Addition of prophylactic medications had begun 3 years ago and she had tried valproic Acid, propranolol, and topiramate without improvement in frequency or intensity of her headaches. She had no comorbid medical or psychiatric conditions. There was no personal family history of alcoholism or substance abuse.

A diagnosis of migraine without aura and MOH was made. She initially underwent outpatient drug withdrawal, and prophylactic treatment with topiramate was initiated. Two weeks later, she was admitted to the neurology ward, and all Triptan medications were stopped. Her withdrawal headache was treated with prednisone and aspirin. During the first 3 days, she suffered a severe migraine attack but was pain-free on day 4. She was discharged on day 5 and asked to keep a headache diary and not take more than 2 doses of the Triptan per week. She returned after 3 months and reported that she was continuing the Topiramate and now had only 2 migraine attacks per month. The diagnosis of MOH was confirmed retrospectively by the fact that the migraine had improved when her Triptan intake was reduced.

Comment

This patient presented with a relatively straightforward diagnosis of MOH and she had no comorbid conditions. Outpatient withdrawal was possible because her overuse drug presented few problems with withdrawal, unlike opioids, barbiturates, or other combination drugs. She also had no medical or psychiatric comorbidities. Some have divided MOH into simple MOH type I or Complex (MOH type II). Simple cases involve short-term drug overuse, modest amounts of overuse of medications, minimal psychiatric contribution, and no history of relapse after drug withdrawal. In contrast, complex cases often present with multiple psychiatric comorbidities and a history of relapse.[26]

Case Report 2

A 40-year-old woman reported suffering from daily headaches. Her migraines had started at the age of 15 years. She had neither aura nor premonitory symptoms. She usually had 1 to 2 migraine attacks per month. During the past 3 to 4 years, the migraine frequency had increased to 5 to 6 attacks per month, each lasting 2 to 3 days. She sometimes treated her migraine attacks with Triptans or Excedrin Migraine, a combination of aspirin, acetaminophen, and caffeine and another containing aspirin and butalbital. Her migraines increased in frequency, and she consequently increased her drug intake until she was taking each medication 15 to 18 days per month. During the last 2 to 3 years, she experienced dull, bilateral headaches in addition to her typical migraine attacks. During the past year, she had taken more headache drugs because of increasing days with bilateral tightening headache. She occasionally borrowed her sister's long-acting opioids but could not remember the exact amount. There was a strong history of substance abuse in her family, and she had been treated within the last year for depression and anxiety. Although alcohol exacerbated her headache frequency and intensity, she occasionally drank 4 to 5 ounces of whiskey "to get away from it all" in spite of the consequences.

She was advised to undergo inpatient drug withdrawal. She developed a withdrawal headache, which was treated for 5 days with prednisone 100 mg. Preventive treatment with topiramate was initiated. A psychiatric consultation was obtained, and she started working with a therapist on her life situation and life style. Intensive education on MOH was begun, and she started a headache and medication diary. Two months later, the patient was experiencing 3 to 4 migraine attacks per month, each lasting 1 to 2 days. Concomitant, dull daily headache disappeared completely.

Comment

This case demonstrates the course of MOH resulting from analgesic, barbiturate, opioid, and/or Triptan overuse. There is some question whether the migraine-like daily headache is more typical with Triptan overuse and tension-type–like daily headache more common with analgesic overuse, but here factors such as barbiturate use, uncertain use of opioids, psychiatric history, and depression mandated inhospital detoxification and management of withdrawal symptoms. It also illustrates that Triptans are expensive and often limited by third-party payers to a certain number per month, usually 9 in the investigators' experience and then patients turn to other agents, often "loosing count" or underestimating the amount they take. After detoxification, a headache and medication diary is imperative. Serious withdrawal phenomena are seen with opioid and barbiturate overuse.

ETIOLOGY AND PATHOPHYSIOLOGY

Medication overuse is obviously the predominant factor in causing MOH but it seems to be unique to headache sufferers. As delineated earlier, chronic use of analgesics for other conditions did not seem to be prone to MOH.[24,25] Risk factors include daily or weekly use of analgesics and more frequent headaches. Low socioeconomic status, immigrant status, obesity, and a positive family history of chronic headache and substance abuse are all risk factors for the development of MOH. As to actual pathophysiology, the sequence of events leading to MOH is largely unknown, but there have been recent studies that she had some light on possible mechanisms. Downregulation of receptors in trigeminal ganglion and, subsequently, a reduction of receptor function have been noted.[27] Chronic administration of 2 Triptans, sumatriptan and zolmitriptan, caused a decrease of the 5-HT synthesis in the dorsal raphe nuclei of the midbrain.[28,29] Triptans given daily resulted in a sensitization of trigeminal nociception, possibly because of increased expression of neuronal nitric oxide synthase in dural afferents. Chronic application of analgesics resulted in upregulation of pronociceptive 5HT2A receptors of platelets in humans, in a significant decrease in the maximum number of 5HT2A binding sites and an increase in the maximum number of 5-HT transporter binding sites in the central nervous system of rats.[30,31]

There is growing evidence showing that central sensitization may play an important role in the pathophysiology of chronic headache. A series of investigations using psychophysical and electrophysiological techniques clearly demonstrated a facilitation of trigeminal pain processing in patients with chronic headache. Decreased pain thresholds have been found in patients with chronic tension-type headache. These findings have been confirmed by demonstrating increased amplitudes of laser-evoked cortical potentials in patients with chronic tension-type headache.[32]

A magnetic resonance imaging (MRI) voxel-based morphometry study revealed structural brainstem changes in patients with chronic tension-type headache but not in patients with MOH.[33] Another study investigated glucose metabolism in 16 patients with MOH before and after withdrawal and in 68 healthy controls. The investigators found reversible hypometabolic changes in brain regions belonging to the general pain network. The orbitofrontal cortex, however, showed persistent hypometabolism before and after drug withdrawal, more so when patients were overusing combination analgesics.[34] In contrast, a recent functional MRI (fMRI) study demonstrated reduced pain-related activity in the pain matrix, which was completely reversible 6 months after withdrawal.[35] MRI voxel-based morphometry and neurophysiological studies such as fMRI in humans and animals will undoubtedly shed light on the phenomena of chronic daily headaches and MOH in the near future.

Genetic studies have generally been ambiguous and unrewarding; psychological factors including fear of headaches, conscious or unconscious fear of withdrawal symptoms also play a role but are difficult to quantify.

PREVENTION

Clearly, the most important factors in the prevention of MOH are the following:

1. Correct diagnosis and familiarizing oneself with the criteria for the diagnosis of episodic migraine without aura (Episodic migraine with aura is usually being much more obvious) and avoiding calling any severe headache a "migraine" and proceeding to treat it as such.
2. Patient education and close follow-up of patients with episodic migraine and tension-type headache, which account for most patients progressing to chronic daily headache and MOH. Unexpected allies are the third-party payers who often restrict the use of Triptans because of cost. However, patients should be carefully instructed to use specific antimigraine drugs for migraine attacks only. The distinction between vasodilating and nondilating headaches was already made in 1951[6] in regard to ergots, and the advice remains fresh today in regard to Triptans and other acute medications for headache.
3. Restricting the number of doses of any kind of acute headache and migraine drugs to 10 doses per month is an effective way to avoid medication overuse. Migraine drugs that contain barbiturates, caffeine, codeine, or tranquilizers, as well as mixed analgesics, should be avoided completely. Patients who take nonprescription medication should be advised to avoid caffeine combinations.
4. Avoidance of chronic Opioid administration.
5. Early migraine prophylaxis with membrane channel blocks, beta-blockers and/or tricyclics or botulinum toxin.
6. Early use of behavioral modification strategies.
7. Headache diaries and medication diaries.

DIFFERENTIAL DIAGNOSIS

Elsewhere in this issue are articles on *The Targeted Headache History* and *Factors which Cause Concern* about headaches. The initial concern in evaluating a new headache patient with frequent headaches, more than 10 to 15 days per month, or one whose pattern of headaches and/or medication use have changed to include headache or medication use for more than 10 to 15 days is whether this is a primary or secondary headache. This is a situation previously alluded to where the classification of MOH causes confusion. The usual secondary headache is one associated with a structural or metabolic lesion of the nervous system, which represents any disabling or potentially lethal condition. MOH represents an intermediate form in which a primary headache type now has a known (although occasionally occult) cause. Often, patients with chronic headaches require reassurance that they do not have a life-threatening condition as an initial step in treatment.

A good understanding of the criteria for the diagnosis of a primary headache type is a necessary first step. However, at all times, it must be borne in mind that increasing medication use may be a result of a secondary condition that is escalating. Indeed, a primary headache may coexist with a secondary headache condition. In a medical practice not specializing in headache care, primary headaches are anticipated to be, by far, the most prevalent ones.

Chronic tension-type headache is a diffuse, dull, nonlocalized headache with or without minimal autonomic features. Headache intensity is lower than that of migraine. Patients find it difficult to describe the character of the pain. Sometimes it is described as a feeling of a metal, rubber, or elastic band around the head or a feeling of increased pressure. Many patients with chronic tension-type headache complain of mild autonomic disturbances such as nausea, photophobia, or phonophobia. Chronic tension-type headache with medication overuse is differentiated from chronic tension-type headache without medication overuse only after drug withdrawal or a drug holiday. If the headache persists, responsibility for chronic headache cannot be attributed to the analgesic intake.

Patients with chronic migraine have a history of episodic migraine attacks that increase in frequency over time. Chronic migraine is diagnosed if patients have daily or almost-daily headaches with migrainous features (eg, unilateral throbbing pain, nausea or vomiting, photophobia and phonophobia, and headache intensity that is increased by physical activity). Most patients are women, 90% of whom have a history of migraine without aura. Chronic migraine has to be distinguished from combination headache, in which patients suffer from chronic tension-type headache along with the daily pressing, tightening, and bilateral headache from intermittent migraine attacks. It is sometimes impossible to separate migraine from tension-type headache. In these cases, treating at least 3 headache days with a Triptan is recommended. If the headache responds to the Triptan, headache prophylaxis is performed as if a migraine exists. The other patients are treated for chronic tension-type headache.

Patients with hemicrania continua suffer from daily headache of moderate intensity. Superimposed exacerbation of severe headache with ipsilateral autonomic features, such as ptosis, miosis, tearing, and sweating may occur. Some patients have photophobia and phonophobia or nausea. In some cases, the head pain alternates sides. Hemicrania continua is differentiated from cluster headache and chronic paroxysmal hemicrania by its continuous pain character; furthermore, the autonomic symptoms during acute pain exacerbations are less pronounced compared with cluster headache or chronic paroxysmal hemicrania.

Patients with new daily persistent headache abruptly develop chronic headache without remission. Many patients remember the exact day the headache started. These patients did not have a previous history of migraine or episodic tension-type headache. In some patients, a viral infection was suspected to cause this form of headache.[36] The headache usually does not respond to ergots, Triptans, or simple analgesics.

The warning signs for secondary headache are covered elsewhere in this issue by the present author, which are briefly enumerated here:

1. Sudden onset of a headache, "the first, worst headache"
2. A worsening headache pattern
3. Headache associated with systemic illness
4. Headache associated with focal neurologic signs
5. Headache associated with personality or cognitive changes
6. Abnormal optic fundus findings

The first step in establishing a diagnosis from the differential diagnosis is a careful history of the headache disorder followed by a thorough general physical and neurologic examination. Then a decision must be made as to further diagnostic laboratory and imaging studies. Frequent acute medication use may be the cause or consequence of the headache disorder. Careful inquiry regarding the course of the headache and acute medication use may suggest chronic migraine when the transformation is gradual over a period of many months or years. An abrupt increase in medication consumption may be caused by a spontaneous increase in the frequency of migraine or tension-type headache. Concomitant medical problems, stress, sleep disturbance, hormonal factors, depression, and certain nonheadache medications can cause an increase in headache frequency.

While there has been substantial objection to imaging of primary headache entities, chronic headaches, especially escalating ones demand thorough workup.

PROGNOSIS

Any attempt to ascertain a prognosis must consider certain factors:

1. What is the definition of success?

Success is defined as no headache at all or an improvement of more than 50% in terms of headache days. The success rate of withdrawal therapy within a time window of the first year is about 70%. Several studies have addressed the long-term outcome of patients with MOH after successful withdrawal therapy.[37–40] Studies with longer observation time of up 6 years reported relapse rates between 40% and 50%.[41–46]

2. Is preventative medication a factor?

Tepper and Tepper[17] give an improvement range of 72% to 85% but bemoan the "preventable relapse" rate listed in various studies.[43,46]

3. What are the predictors for relapse?

Predictors for relapses after successful withdrawal therapy remain difficult to analyze. Two aspects appear to be important: the type of primary headache (patients with tension-type headache or co-occurrence of migraine and tension-type headache have a higher relapse risk)[39,41] and a longer duration of regular drug intake.

4. Is there a significant difference in outcome at 1 year with inpatient versus outpatient treatment?

There does not appear to be a significant difference in these 2 approaches.[47]

5. Is there a difference between abrupt and gradual withdrawal?

There are no studies comparing gradual and abrupt interruption of medication but there is a widespread opinion that drug withdrawal is more effective when done abruptly because this is believed to achieve a fast resolution of the drug-induced pain-coping behavior.[12]

TREATMENT

Abrupt drug withdrawal is the treatment of choice for medication overuse headache. Although there are no studies comparing gradual and abrupt interruption, the widespread opinion of specialists considers drug withdrawal to be more effective when done abruptly because this is believed to achieve a fast resolution of the drug-induced pain-coping behavior.

Most drugs causing MOH can be stopped abruptly. This is most particular to the overuse of Triptans, ergots, paracetamol (acetaminophen), aspirin, and NSAIDs. However, because of the possibility of severe withdrawal symptoms, gradual withdrawal is appropriate with opioids, barbiturates, and, in particular, benzodiazepines. As with drugs that produce a withdrawal syndrome, gradual reduction in caffeine intake may be preferable to abrupt withdrawal."[12]

Withdrawal symptoms last for 2 to 10 days (average 3.5 days) and include withdrawal headache, nausea, vomiting, hypotension, tachycardia, sleep disturbances, restlessness, anxiety, and nervousness. Shorter withdrawal times are observed in MOH patients who are abusing only Triptans. Seizures or hallucinations were only rarely observed, even in patients who were abusing barbiturate-containing migraine drugs. Fluids should be replaced by infusion if frequent vomiting occurs. Vomiting can be treated with antiemetics (eg, metoclopramide or domperidone). The withdrawal headache can be treated with NSAIDs (eg, naproxen 500 mg twice daily). In some countries, aspirin is available in injectable form and 1000 mg is given every 8 to 12 hours. If the headache has migrainous features and the patient has not abused ergotamine, intravenous dihydroergotamine 1 to 2 mg every 8 hours is given. Symptoms of opioid withdrawal can be treated with clonidine. The initial dose is 0.1 to 0.2 mg 3 times daily, and this is titrated up or down based on withdrawal symptoms (tachycardia, tremor, sleeping disturbances). Some patients may require anxiolytic medication; this should be given for no longer than a week.

The question of the relative efficacy of inpatient versus outpatient withdrawal protocols has been alluded to under *prognosis* in this article. Suffice it to repeat that there appears to be no difference in outcome measures. A consensus paper by the German Migraine Society recommends outpatient withdrawal for highly motivated patients who do not take barbiturates or tranquilizers with their analgesics.[48] Patients who take tranquilizers, codeine, or barbiturates and who failed to withdraw the drugs as outpatients or who have a high depression score should have inpatient treatment.[12] Other recent studies demonstrated that psychological education alone is equally effective as a cognitive behavioral contact program and that a team approach is warranted.[42,49] Outpatient withdrawal in uncomplicated patients with MOH is suggested.[12] Patients with psychiatric or psychological comorbidities should be treated using a multidisciplinary treatment approach.[49,50]

There is no unanimity of approach to drug withdrawal in different studies. Measures include fluid replacement, analgesics, tranquilizers, neuroleptics, amitriptyline, valproate, intravenous dihydroergotamine, oxygen, and electrical stimulation. There has been a tendency to use prednisone or its congeners to alleviate withdrawal symptoms, but studies on cortisone to reduce withdrawal headache are ambiguous. In an editorial in 2007, Diener[21] reviewed the evidence to date and concluded that "The first open trial showed that treatment of the withdrawal symptoms of MOH requires higher doses of prednisone or prednisolone; corticosteroids are only effective in migraine patients with MOH and not in patients with tension type headache; and using prednisone in open trials provokes a high placebo response." When used, a typical regimen is prednisone 100 mg on the first day, tapering by 20 mg per day until weaned.

A small pilot placebo-controlled study in Germany demonstrated the superiority of oral prednisone 100 mg versus placebo.[51] Another larger study from Norway, however, produced negative result for relief from withdrawal symptoms with prednisolone.[38]

Another issue is starting a prophylactic medication, especially for migraine sufferers. Tepper and Tepper[17] state that the prophylactic regimen can be started before or during the weaning from the overused medication, whereas Negro and Martelletti,[12] emphasizing chronic migraine as the most frequent inciting headache type for MOH advocate prophylactic therapy for all patients with more than 3 disabling attacks per month despite the "appropriate use" of acute medications.[52,53] Topiramate and onabotulinum toxin A are advocated by Tepper and Tepper.[17] They cite studies of topiramate in which topiramate was proved to be effective in reducing migraine headache days[54–56] and able to reduce the risk of transformation to a chronic form.[56] The most common adverse events during topiramate treatment are paresthesias (8%), cognitive symptoms (7.3%), fatigue (4.7%), insomnia (3.4%), nausea (2.3%), loss of appetite, anxiety, and dizziness (2.1%). They advocate[17] onabotulinum toxin A even more strongly o a lower side effect profile, based on the PREEMPT 1 and PREEMPT 2 studies.[57–59]

Patients who have chronic tension-type headache may be started on a tricyclic antidepressant 4 weeks before detoxification (eg, amitriptyline, 10 mg, increasing to 25 to 75 mg at nighttime).

When evaluating chronic headache patients, it is necessary to take a careful history. These patients frequently take several different substances daily despite the fact that their effect is negligible. This behavior is merely an attempt to avoid a disabling withdrawal headache. Patients should record their present and prior use of prescription drugs and nonprescription compounds and caffeine intake. Many patients also abuse other substances, such as tranquilizers, opioids, decongestants, and laxatives. It is often helpful for patients to keep a diagnostic headache diary for 1 month to actually record headache patterns and drug use. History and examination should also search for possible complications of regular drug intake, such as recurrent gastric ulcers, anemia, and ergotism.

Measures other than pharmacology may be helpful.[50] Patients need the support of treating physicians and nurses as well as encouragement from family and friends. Behavioral techniques, such as relaxation therapy and stress management, should be initiated as soon as the withdrawal symptoms fade. Headache school, headache nurses, physical therapists, and psychologists all have a role in specialized headache clinics, that is, a "team approach."[50] Again, outcome measures are difficult to obtain, vary from study to study, due in large part to selection of different outcome parameters.

SUMMARY

"An ounce of prevention is worth a pound of cure" in the management of MOH. Prevention of transformation of primary headache types to their chronic counterparts is necessary to prevent this most troubling transformation. Strict attention to what patients are telling you (and often times not telling you) about their episodic headaches will enable pharmacologic and nonpharmacologic measures to avoid that transformation to chronic daily headache, so often associated with MOH. Once MOH becomes manifest, withdrawal of the overused drug is mandatory; otherwise experience tells us the pattern of overuse will only be perpetuated and no measure will help alleviate the headache. At the same time, as detoxification takes place, measures to ensure that relapse will not take place should begin. These efforts include prophylactic pharmacologic measures as well as psychological support, education, and surveillance to prevent relapses. The rate of relapse is unfortunately high, but these general and specific measures enumerated above will add greatly to the chances of success.

REFERENCES

1. Diener HC, Limmroth V. Medication-overuse headache: a worldwide problem. Lancet Neurol 2004;3:475–83.

2. Headache Classification Committee of the International Headache Society. The international classification of headache disorders. Cephalalgia 2004;24(Suppl 1): 1–160.

3. Olesen J, Lipton RB. Headache classification update 2004. Curr Opin Neurol 2004;17:275–82.

4. Olesen J, Bousser MG, Diener HC, et al. New appendix criteria open for a broader concept of chronic migraine. Cephalalgia 2006;26:742–6.

5. Horton BT, Peters GA. Clinical manifestations of excessive use of ergotamine preparations and management of withdrawal effect: report of 52 cases. Headache 1963;3:214–26.

6. Peters GA, Horton BT. Headache: with special reference to the excessive use of ergotamine preparations and withdrawal effects. Proc Staff Meet Mayo Clin 1951; 26:153–61.

7. Isler H. Headache drugs provoking chronic headache: historical aspects and common misunderstandings. In: Diener HC, Wildinson M, editors. Drug-induced headache. New York, London, Paris, Tokyo: Springer-Verlag Berlin Heidelberg; 1988. p. 87–93.

8. Headache Classification Committee of the International Headache Society. Classification and diagnostic criteria for headache disorders, cranial neuralgia, and facial pain. Cephalalgia 1988;8:1–96.

9. Silberstein SD, Lipton RB, Sliwinski M. Classification of daily and near-daily headaches: field trial of revised IHS criteria. Neurology 1996;47:871–5.

10. Diener HC, Silberstein S. Medication overuse headache. In: Olesen J, Goadsby PJ, Ramadan N, et al, editors. The headaches. Philadelphia: Lippincott Williams Wilkins; 2006. p. 475–83.

11. Lenaerts ME, Couch JR. Medication overuse headache. Minerva Med 2007;98: 221–31.

12. Negro A, Martelletti P. Chronic migraine plus medication overuse headache: two entities or not? J Headache Pain 2011;12:593–601.

13. Couch JR, Lenaerts ME. Medication overuse headache: clinical features, pathogenesis and management. Drug Dev Res 2007;68:1–12.

14. Olesen J, Bousser MG, Diener H, et al. The international classification of headache disorders, 2nd edn. Cephalalgia 2004;24(Suppl 1):1–160.

15. Rapoport A, Weeks R, Sheftell F. Analgesic rebound headache: theoretical and practical implications. In: Olesen J, Tfelt-Hansen P, Jensen K, editors. Proceedings second international headache congress. Copenhagen (Denmark): Kopenhagen; 1985. p. 448–9.

16. Limmroth V, Kazarawa S, Fritsche G, et al. Features of medication overuse headache following overuse of different acute headache drugs. Neurology 2002;59:1011–4.

17. Tepper SJ, Tepper DE. Breaking the cycle of medication overuse headache. Cleve Clin J Med 2010;77:236–42.

18. Bigal ME, Serrano D, Buse D, et al. Acute migraine medications and evolution from episodic to chronic migraine: a longitudinal population based study. Headache 2008;48:1157–68.

19. Diener HC, Dahlof CG. Headache associated with chronic use of substances. In: Olesen J, Tfelt-Hansen P, Welch KM, editors. The headaches. 2nd edition. Philadelphia: Lippincott, Williams & Wilkins; 1999. p. 871–8.

20. Zeeberg P, Olesen J, Jensen R. Probable medication-overuse headache: the effect of a 2-month drug-free period. Neurology 2006;66:1894–8.

21. Diener HC. How to treat medication overuse headache prednisolone or no prednisolone? [editorials]. Neurology 2007;69:14–5.

22. Scher AI, Stewart WF, Ricci JA, et al. Factors associated with the onset and remission of chronic daily headache in a population-based study. Pain 2003; 106:81–9.

23. Katsarava Z, Schneeweiss S, Kurth T, et al. Incidence and predictors for chronicity of headache in patients with episodic migraine. Neurology 2004;62:788–90.

24. Bahra A, Walsh M, Menon S, et al. Does chronic daily headache arise de novo in association with regular analgesic use? Headache 2003;43:179–90.

25. Lance F, Parkes C, Wilkinson M. Does analgesic abuse cause headache de novo? Headache 1988;38:61–2.

26. Mehlsteibel D, Schankin C, Hering P, et al. Anxiety disorders in headache patient's in a specialised clinic: prevalence and symptoms in comparison to patients in a general neurological clinic. J Headache Pain 2011;12:323–9.

27. Reuter U, Salomone S, Ickstein GW, et al. Effects of chronic sumatriptan and zolmitriptan treatment on 5-HAT receptor expression and function in rats. Cephalalgia 2004;24:398–407.

28. Dobson CF, Tohyama Y, Diksic M, et al. Effects of acute or chronic administration of anti-migraine drugs sumatriptan and zolmitriptan on serotonin synthesis in the rat brain. Cephalalgia 2004;24:2–11.

29. Tohyama Y, Yamane F, Fikre Merid M, et al. Effects of serotonin receptor agonists, TFMPP and CGS12066B, on regional serotonin synthesis in the rat brain: an autoradiographic study. J Neurochem 2002;80:788–98.

30. Srikiatkhachorn A, Anthony M. Platelet serotonin in patients with analgesic-induced headache. Cephalalgia 1996;16(6):423–6.

31. Srikiatkhachorn A, Tarasub N, Govitrapong P. Effect of chronic analgesic exposure on the central serotonin system: a possible mechanism of analgesic abuse headache. Headache 2000;40(5):343–50.

32. de Tommaso M, Libro G, Guido M, et al. Heat pain thresholds and cerebral event-related potentials following painful CO_2 laser stimulation in chronic tension-type headache. Pain 2003;104:111–9.

33. Schmidt-Wilcke T, Leinisch E, Straube A, et al. Gray matter decrease in patients with chronic tension type headache. Neurology 2005;65:1483–6.

34. Fumal A, Laureys S, Di Clemente L, et al. Orbitofrontal cortex involvement in chronic analgesic-overuse headache evolving from episodic migraine. Brain 2006;129:543–50.

35. Ferraro S, Grazzi L, Mandelli ML, et al. Pain processing in medication overuse headache: a functional magnetic resonance imaging (fMRI) study. Pain Med 2012;13(2):255–62.

36. Diaz-Mitoma F, Vanast WJ, Tyrrell DL. Increased frequency of Epstein-Barr-virus excretion in patients with new daily persistent headaches. Lancet 1987;1(8530): 411–4.

37. Baumgartner C, Wessely P, Bingol C, et al. Long-term prognosis of analgesic withdrawal in patients with drug-induced headaches. Headache 1989;29:510–4.

38. Boe MG, Mygland A, Salvesen R. Prednisolone does not reduce withdrawal headache: a randomized, double-blind study. Neurology 2007;69(1):26–31.

39. Diener HC, Dichgans J, Scholz E, et al. Analgesic-induced chronic headache: long-term results of withdrawal therapy. J Neurol 1989;236:9–14.

40. Grazzi L, Andrasik F, D'Amico D, et al. Behavioral and pharmacologic treatment of transformed migraine with analgesic overuse: outcome at 3 years. Headache 2002;42:483–90.

41. Evers S, Suhr B, Bauer B, et al. A retrospective long-term analysis of the epidemiology and features of drug-induced headache. Neurology 1999;246(9):802–9.

42. Fritsche G, Frettlööh J, Hüppe M, et al. Prevention of medication overuse in patients with migraine. Pain 2010;15(2):404–13.
43. Pini LA, Cicero AF, Sandrini M. Long-term follow-up of patients treated for chronic headache with analgesic overuse. Cephalalgia 2001;21(9):878–83.
44. Schnider P, Aull S, Baumgartner C, et al. Long-term outcome of patients with headache and drug abuse after inpatient withdrawal: five year follow-up. Cephalalgia 1996;16:481–5.
45. Tribl GG, Schnider P, Wober C, et al. Are there predictive factors for long-term outcome after withdrawal in drug-induced chronic daily headache? Cephalalgia 2001;21(6):691–6.
46. Zidverc-Trajkovic J, Pekmezovic T, Jovanovic Z, et al. Medication overuse headache: clinical features predicting treatment outcome at 1-year follow-up. Cephalalgia 2007;27(11):1219–25.
47. Grazzi L, Andrasik F, Usai S, et al. In-patient versus day- hospital withdrawal treatment for chronic migraine with medication overuse and disability assessment: results one year followup. Neurol Sci 2008;29:161–3.
48. Diener HC, Evers S, Fritsche G, et al. Medication overuse headache. In: Diener HC, editor. Guidelines of the german society of neurology. Thieme Verlag; 2009.
49. Gaul C, van Doorn C, Webering N, et al. Clinical outcome of a headache-specific multidisciplinary treatment program and adherence to treatment recommendations in a tertiary headache center: an observational study. J Headache Pain 2011;12:475–83.
50. Gaul C, Visscher CM, Bhola R, et al. Team players against headache: multidisciplinary treatment of primary headaches and medication overuse headache. J Headache Pain 2011;12:511–9.
51. Pageler L, Katsarava Z, Diener HC, et al. Prednisone vs. placebo in withdrawal therapy following medication overuse headache. Cephalalgia 2008;28(2):152–6.
52. Lipton RB, Bigal ME, Diamond M, et al. Migraine prevalence, disease burden, and the need for preventive therapy. Neurology 2007;68:343–9.
53. Antonaci F, Dumitrache C, De Cillis I, et al. A review of current European guidelines for migraine. J Headache Pain 2010;11:13–9.
54. Diener HC, Bussone G, Van Oene JC, et al, TOPMAT-MIG-201(TOP-CHROME) Study Group. Topiramate reduces headache days in chronic migraine: a randomized, double-blind, placebo-controlled study. Cephalalgia 2007;27:814–23.
55. Silberstein SD, Lipton RB, Dodick DW, et al, Group Topiramate Chronic Migraine Study. Efficacy and safety of topiramate for the treatment of chronic migraine: a randomized, double-blind, placebo-controlled trial. Headache 2007;47:170–80.
56. Silberstein SD, Neto W, Schmitt J, et al, MIGR-001 Study Group. Topiramate in migraine prevention: results of a large controlled trial. Arch Neurol 2004;61:490–5.
57. Dodick DW, Turkel CC, DeGryse RE, et al, PREEMPT Chronic Migraine Study Group. OnabotulinumtoxinA for treatment of chronic migraine: pooled results from the double-blind, randomized placebo-controlled phases of the PREEMPT clinical program. Headache 2010;50:921–36.
58. Aurora SK, Dodick DW, Turkel CC, et al, PREEMPT 1 Chronic Migraine Study Group. OnabotulinumtoxinA for treatment of chronic migraine: results from the double-blind, randomized placebo-controlled phase of the PREEMPT 1 trial. Cephalalgia 2010;30:793–803.
59. Diener HC, Dodick DW, Aurora SK, et al, PREEMPT 2 Chronic Migraine Study Group. OnabotulinumtoxinA for treatment of chronic migraine: results from the double-blind, randomized, placebo-controlled phase of the PREEMPT 2 trial. Cephalalgia 2010;30:804–14.

Index

Note: Page numbers of article titles are in **boldface** type.

Med Clin N Am 97 (2013) 353–362
http://dx.doi.org/10.1016/S0025-7125(13)00012-6
0025-7125/13/$ – see front matter © 2013 Elsevier Inc. All rights reserved.

medical.theclinics.com

Moving?

Make sure your subscription moves with you!

To notify us of your new address, find your **Clinics Account Number** (located on your mailing label above your name), and contact customer service at:

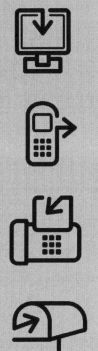

Email: journalscustomerservice-usa@elsevier.com

800-654-2452 (subscribers in the U.S. & Canada)
314-447-8871 (subscribers outside of the U.S. & Canada)

Fax number: 314-447-8029

Elsevier Health Sciences Division
Subscription Customer Service
3251 Riverport Lane
Maryland Heights, MO 63043

Printed and bound by CPI Group (UK) Ltd, Croydon, CR0 4YY

13/10/2024

01773580-0001